The Life Sensei's Guide

2

I0454788

Health

Cover Art and Interior Design by Terence Mitchell

Copyright© 2014 by Terence Mitchell

Printed in the USA

Dedication

I would like to dedicate this book to my clients, new and old, who challenge me to put forth my best. I hope it finds new readers open-minded and adventurous. I am amazed at your ability to come every week and shape your future. For anyone exposed to the "Trained" mentality for the first time, welcome aboard!

To my mother who has continued to amaze me and show me that there is never a time to abandon what you believe in. I will always be proud of you, and will be always in your cheering section. I love you.

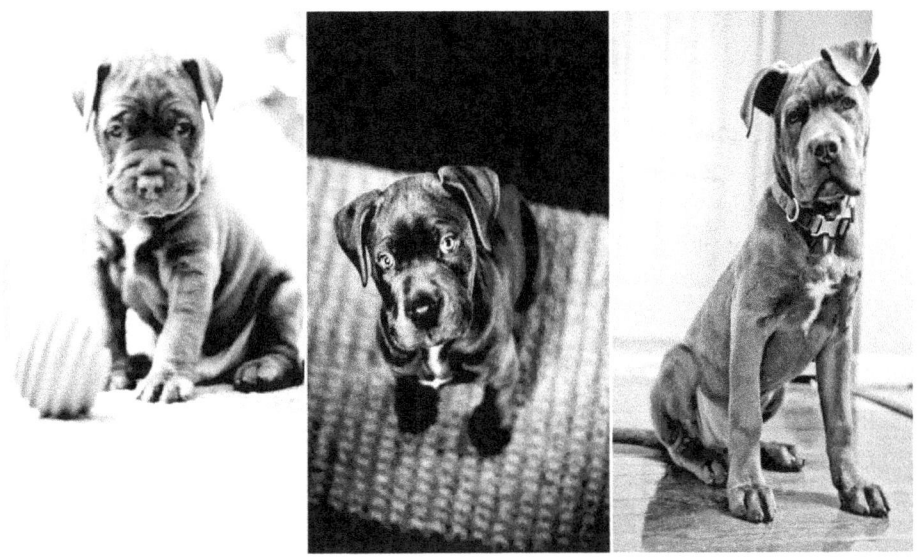

Thor you have brought me
immeasurable joy!

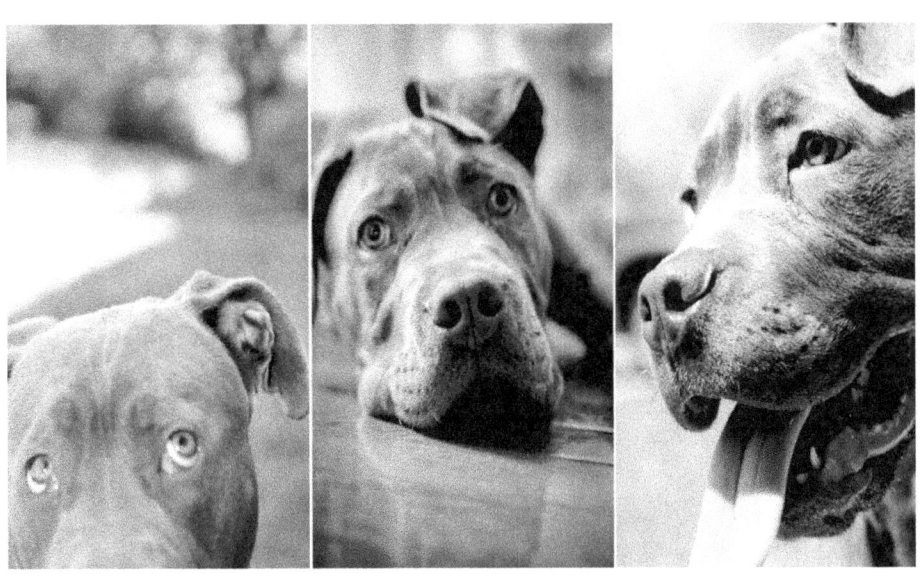

Acknowledgements

First and foremost, I want to give all glory to GOD. I pray this book reaches people's hearts and changes lives. In GOD all things are possible. I pray I can be used by You however You see fit. Thanks for the words, You are my ROCK.

Thank you to the Artistic Journalist Publishing Team for your invaluable help editing the book. Thanks to all the others that helped me shape this book through conversation, experiences, and thanks to all the models that allowed themselves to shine through my camera.

There are too many people to list who have helped me develop as a person, thus contributing to this book. I have the fortune of calling these people friends. You know who you are. Thanks for the love, wisdom and support.

Foreword

As children, almost everyone has desires, hopes, and dreams. Many things in life affect whether these future expectations are reached. There are objectives to reach goals, usually set into motion by planning and may unfold as luck and/or blessing or both. When you become a parent you want your child to be healthy, you want that child to have every opportunity in the world to become what they want to be and yes, you hope no harm will come to them. In the meantime the parent does their best to instill values, self-worth, respect for others, and a sense of independence in their child so that they can manage and take care of themselves. But then you realize as a parent that your child has desires, hopes, and dreams of their own. They have to go through the obstacles of life to get where they want to go.

You know as a parent that you cannot protect your child from everything. You can only hope that they will find their way with very few hurts and scars. Yet, you hope that your child will grow in wisdom, truth, and a sense of self and treat others fairly and with respect. Although you know as a parent, and a "former child", that this ability only comes with a measurement of pain, gain, and disappointments.

You hope they can love and cherish and carry on the wealth of love, positive belief, and appropriate generosity. You want them to do well in school, obtain a good salary from their work, and share the wealth of a life lived with good intentions. This book is a great snapshot of a life lived with the wealth of love, hurt, redemption, the pouring out of experiences lived, lessons learned, and a need to connect with others to improve their lives.

Become love-wealthy

Enjoy,

Giselle K. Mitchell (in the role of mom)

How to Use This Book

There is A LOT of information in this book and it must be read repeatedly to obtain its true value. My intention is to give relevant information to those who need it so they may apply, understand, and ultimately share it with others. Feel free to flip through the book as needed or read it chapter by chapter. This book is about becoming **your personal best**. Everybody who reads this will interpret things differently.

My philosophy as a teen was always somewhat confusing to me. I have never fully understood why I think and behave the way I do. As an adult, my philosophy has driven me to change the things that I didn't like about myself; I (with GOD's help) have attempted to change for the better. Now as a Sensei, my philosophy is motivated by simpler things. I am motivated by seeing others succeed, grow and become truly happy. As a result, I succeed, grow and become happy as well. I can sum it up best by stating:

"My Philosophy is to live life with love, to care for others, and learn to understand what makes us different; to truly believe in yourself, think past problems and setbacks". Accomplish your goals and excel in life while enjoying the process; become the best you possible."

Are you TRAINED to be the best *YOU* possible?

Throughout this book you will see these words repeatedly. They are meant to help you better understand a philosophy that has changed my world and hopefully will help change yours. My Sensei used to say, "You can't master someone's body until you master your own."I now also believe, "You can't master understanding others until you understand yourself".

Contents:

"Reflect on what you see daily, apply what you reflect on and never stop learning." -Sensei Mitchell aka the Life Sensei

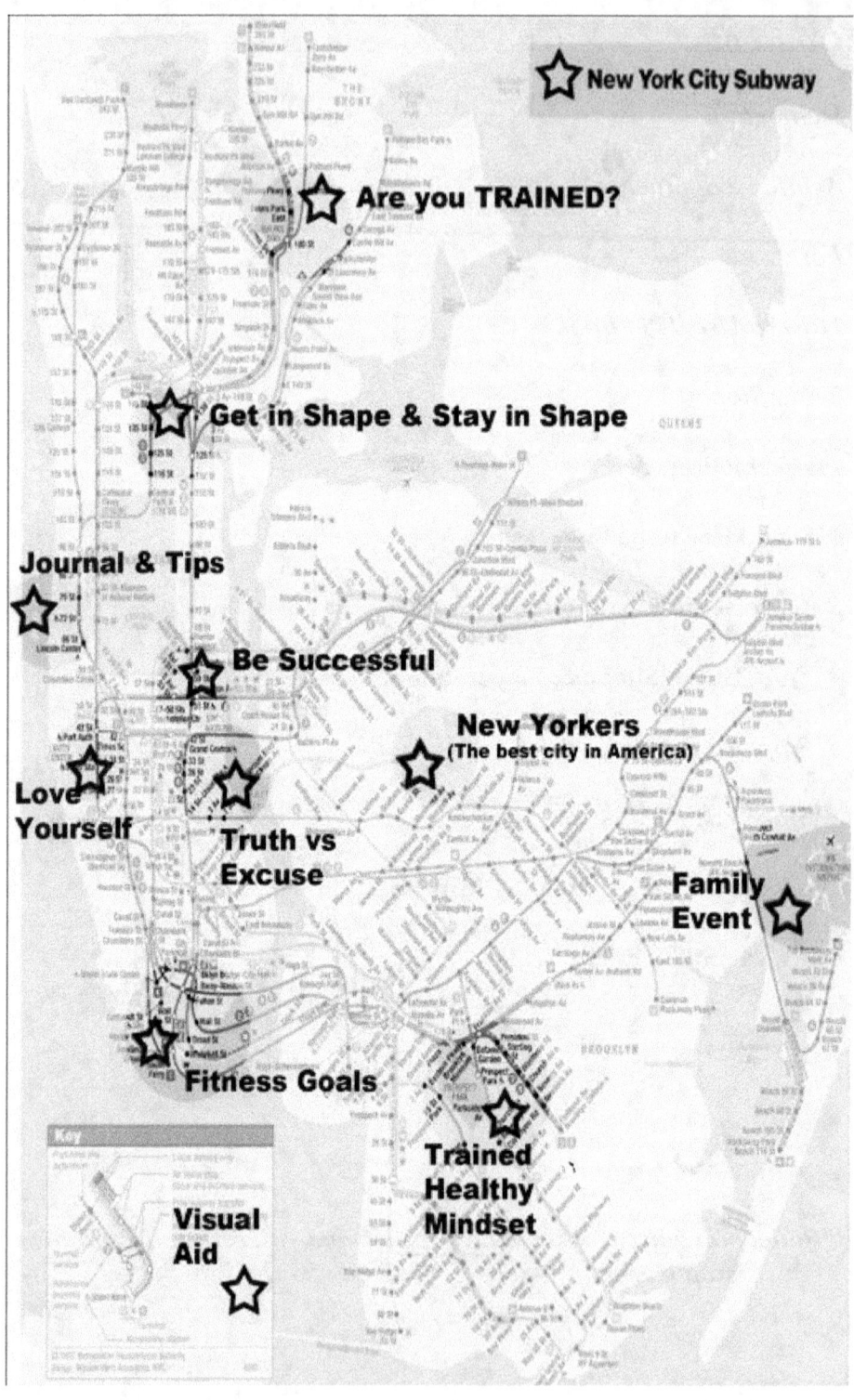

☆ New York City Subway

☆ Are you TRAINED?

☆ Get in Shape & Stay in Shape

Journal & Tips
☆

☆ Be Successful

New Yorkers
☆ (The best city in America)

☆
Love
Yourself

☆ Truth vs
Excuse

Family
Event ☆

☆ Fitness Goals

☆ Trained
Healthy
Mindset

Visual
Aid
☆

Wake up & Warm up
5 head circles in each direction
10 arm swings
1:30 jog in place
20 high knees
2 jump squats
5 side lunges each side
5 squat thrusts
30 kick backs
20 standing calf raises
2:00 standing hamstring strecth
1:00 calf stretch each leg
:15 tricep stretch each arm
shake it out

theLifeSenSei.trainerze.com for the videos to exercises

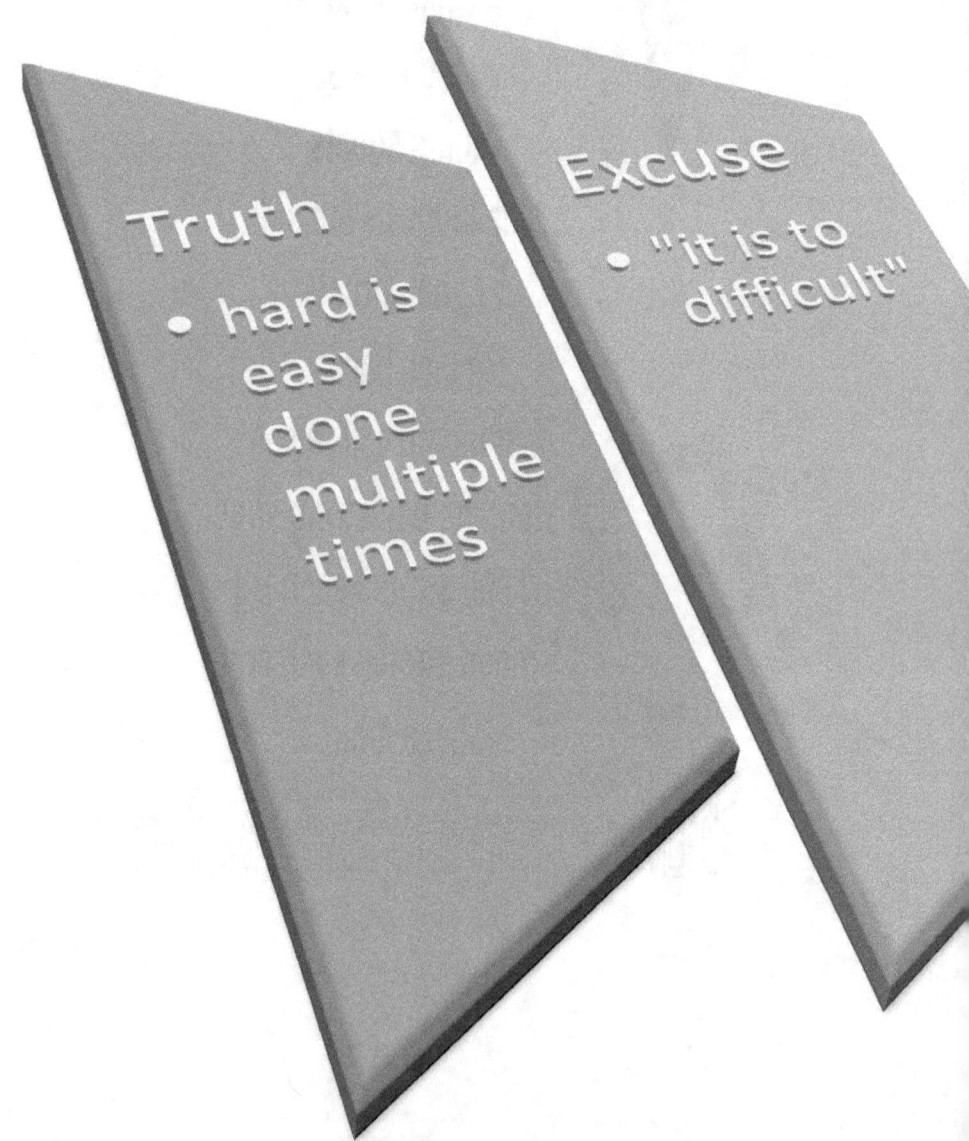

"Planning" Advice

Here you are going to find general tips

To get you going and keep you informed,

Could be fun, serious, noteworthy

Enjoy!

"Implement" Means Business

Here is 100% Coach "T" advice

These are non-negotiable

So apply these to your life and "invest" in yourself

Good "Habits" Help You Focus

This is where you will find info to help you

Meditate: find your center and balance

Are You "Results" Oriented?

This is where I am going to push you

Take you further than you are comfortable going

Are you going to push back?

www.trained2b.com

Platform: Preface

I have always been passionate about life, its ups and downs, highs and lows. Life has a way of keeping you on your toes, always "offering" surprises and new experiences. There is no other city in the world which best represents life than New York City. Growing up in New York City is in some ways different than growing up anywhere else. It is sink or swim, and in NYC, you learn to swim fast. Some people might say there are many obstacles stopping you from succeeding in life. I'd like to think of it as there being many hurdles. Are you ready to jump? In life, we must learn to deal with situations new and old decisively, so we make the most of opportunities.

I thank GOD for the opportunities available to kids back then. Even though it was crazy, people looked out for one another; neighborhoods were safer. I was not just my mom's kid; I had a whole neighborhood of parents. I'm talking about a melting pot of parents, who all looked out for us. That was an admirable thing, although it might not have felt that way then. As a child, I was disciplined for acting up and doing the wrong thing. Today I cannot understand how people can be so spoiled and lack manners. Children yelling at parents and getting whatever they want. I digress.

Riding the buses, subways, and surviving by trial and error on the streets of New York at a young age is still common. My father and mother enjoyed three years of happy marriage and celebrated the arrival of twin sons born in Harlem. (She thought she was going to have one son and was blessed with two).

As the years passed, my mom became a single parent. I am pleased to say that she set an extraordinary example for being a strong, goal oriented, GOD fearing woman. I would not trade the way I was raised, even if growing up was not easy. I believe that everything in life happens for a reason and I am comfortable with that. Whatever my father's reasons, I am grateful that he did not complicate our lives with negativity. I hear horror stories of fathers who are one foot out the door raising their kids with confusion, mistrust and a lack of love. I did not realize how a father can play a significant role in a child's life until much later in mine.

Things that many men take for granted I found as an adult I could have used. I am amazed to meet people that do not use the skills they were taught at an earlier age. The insight I gained from being raised primarily by women has helped separate me from the wolf pack in my personal and business endeavors.

My mother worked, went to school and raised two boys with my grandmother's help. As latch key children, my brother and I had to fend for ourselves at a young age. We fought quite a bit, starting as young boys in elementary school to men in college. My brother was my first sparring partner. Though he drives me crazy, I love him dearly. I was an unsightly kid with a big belly, glasses, skinny as a twig and fast as lightning. I was taught the value of an education, so I was called a nerd. If it was not for the Boys and Girls Club, an afterschool program designed to educate and keep children off the street, I do not know where my brother and I might have ended up. My passion for fitness started pretty much like anybody else. Being young, shy and book smart, I was naive to the benefits of being athletic. I could play ping pong, pool, table tennis or board games better than most, but sports were a privilege for lucky or wealthier kids. I loved watching action and martial art movies as a kid, and I longed to become a hero just like the ones I watched on the big screen. When the opportunity arrived, I began taking a self-defense class at the Boys Club when I was twelve years old. My interest in Martial Arts and fitness has continued to this day.

You might wonder why I go through all this trouble to talk about NYC. What does a book about fitness and becoming your personal best have to do with a city? I think it is essential to use examples, I believe that you will retain the material and apply it better if you can relate. What better city in the world than NYC to compare our lives to? New Yorkers are spread throughout the world. Chances are you have come across one in your life (like the fabled unicorn). Your family might have immigrated here. You might even have been born and/or raised here; the truth is we are all, like it or not, New Yorkers. A New Yorker is someone who does not quit, who continues to strive, who when faced with adversity rises to the occasion. Like a train rising from underground looking over the city streets, speeding along its course, we are all looking to elevate our status, lifestyle, or position. When our city was attacked as a country we united under the banner of New York. As a country we all related. We were all New Yorkers.

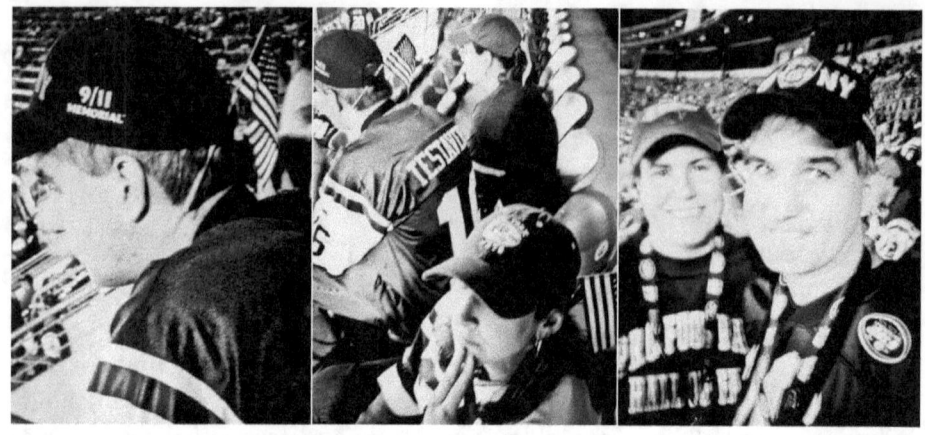

In regards to fitness, in New York, it may appear you are only in shape as long as you need to be. Many people work out so that they can say they work out; working out to look good, not because it is healthy. We work out because that is what society has coined a trend. Do not be fooled by the whole fitness craze; society contains people who have invested many dollars on diet products and memberships to gyms who never set foot in them. Most people want to be healthy, but claim they do not have the resources, fortitude, or time.

In New York, if being heavy set was the style tomorrow everybody would start doing it today. I am aware there are health conscious people out there and that I am generalizing, but this is the reality for many people. We go with the tide in NYC, and the high tide is in right now so fashionably fit is how we roll. So are the Knickerbockers, healthy choice menus, super hero movies and social media. Trans-fat is out, so are cigarettes, 42nd street, free parking spots, low medical bills and cheap concert tickets.

Back in the day, it did not matter about your shape or style. No one cared whether you shopped at Macy's or a thrift store. I used to wear cheap clothing before it was fashionable, it was probably laughable, but it did not stop me. People accepted themselves for who they were and did not pay attention to what others thought as much as people do now. That is part of the reason people are so insecure about their bodies and self-image, living according to what others believe is cool, real and all that nonsense.

Your family teaches you that you're unique and valuable. As you begin to interact with the rest of the world, you learned that not everyone will feel that way about you. So you have a choice, conform and replicate what is already out there or be yourself, unique and different. Unfortunately, many choose the former. The insecurity comes in when you feel like you're being pulled from all directions and do not know who you are. In New York, there are simply more people, more opportunities, more experiences and more life lessons.

You would be amazed at all the things you learn in New York on a daily basis; the kindness of strangers and the seemingly rude behavior of people. You learn about the areas you can and cannot hang out at for safety. You learn that not everyone has the same views as yours. The lesson that the world is much bigger than you and you should not put all your hopes and dreams in sports, music, or the lottery becomes apparent. You learn that people die of old age but, in New York, many people die from unnatural causes. You learn that New York is governed by money and coming in a close second, time.

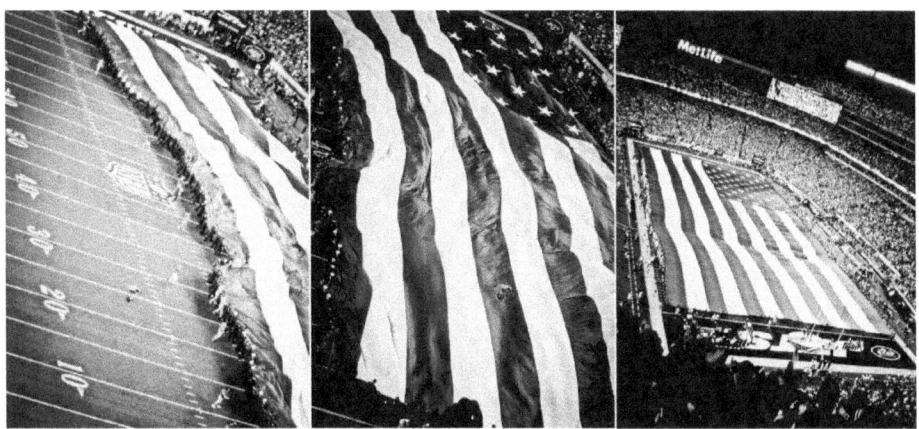

Everyone is connected one way or another. In life, you have many opportunities to learn about diversity and the lack of respect there is for people that are different. Many people believe in a higher power, some call it the almighty dollar. Others call it a gun, drugs and or the opposite sex. I grew up thinking I knew everything as typical as any teen. Thanks to my Mom I knew the Village (in the lower part of Manhattan) like the back of my hand, and used to laugh when the older kids would play hooky to hang out there and get lost.

I was exposed to the club scene when I was sixteen and partied underage for free. My friends and I laughed while people would drive an hour and pay through the nose to stand outside on a long line, wondering if they were going to get inside the clubs. That exposure helped me grow up fast and although the beginning of my life was not the way I planned it, I am grateful for the life lessons learned.

When I first obtained the ranking of Sensei it was a title to go along with my job, the weight of the responsibility did not hit me until later. When you see teachers it is easy to believe that all they do is instruct on a subject. Teachers are skilled communicators, sharing their knowledge in a way that resonates with their students. They have to be willing to want comprehensive students, who can duplicate and apply what they learn. Teachers inspire you to learn about life. New York City was an excellent teacher. I teach how to survive, develop a warrior's instinct, skill sets and become a better prepared, better in shape you. It is now something I continuously aspire to, a goal to develop myself to the best of my abilities.

As my students reap the rewards of their hard efforts, I feel alive. Why are these skill sets prudent? I learned you could not always win arguments or battles with words, sometimes you had to defend yourself. If you "defended" yourself too well you could get in more trouble; get jumped, have legal woes, do time in jail or worse, answer to the wrath of your parents. I learned getting drunk was not fun in my teens. I learned that just because you're honest does not mean everyone will appreciate it.

I moved out when I was a teen thinking that I could do better without my family. (I moved back in shortly after). I've witnessed people destroy their lives with drugs, and end their lives before they started. I've seen friends lives cut short because they were at the wrong place. This is normal to a New Yorker, day to day, becoming hardened to experiences and relationships. I was 16, living in Brooklyn with a full time job. I paid my own rent but, something was missing. I did what I could to make money as honestly as possible. I worked as a delivery person, fast food cook (do not eat the eggs), supermarket associate, dental assistant, camp counselor, stock person, and sneaker salesman all before I was eighteen. I guess it surprises me when people refuse to work certain jobs or choose not to work at all.

I stayed true to the streets and navigated through them like a native of the concrete jungle. I played my position well and was respected because of it, but inside I was empty.

In New York, you also learned that a bullet has no name on it and that no one is promised tomorrow. Getting robbed at the sneaker store changed my outlook on life. I found purpose at church and I learned about GOD. I moved home with a better understanding of my family. I returned to school and earned the title of salutatorian. The value of continuing my education and doing more for myself and others nagged at me. I studied Pastoral Ministry and Philosophy at college. I always wanted to be part of something that gave back to the community, though I did not always know why. I struggled with the concept of not being able to reach those who would not attend the church. I believe that our future can only be assured if we give and receive with open hearts.

Trained 2 B Tip

"Tough moments will never last, tough people do"

My job experience in retail as a teen afforded me a career in management, which I disliked. I enjoyed my employees and the clients, but the pretense in running stores for profit vs. caring for the customer was too much for me. I always envisioned being fortunate to work for myself and live the life I always wanted. Being able to make my own schedule has its benefits, as well as, the time to pursue the hobbies and dreams I enjoy. Sometimes being your own boss means less financial gain, but I will always trade the money for my happiness. As I slowly matured, like a lamb becoming a sheep, I learned to play fair and do what I had to survive. I have always loved the school where I trained, and when the opportunity presented itself; I did not hesitate in taking over the school and following my dreams. It is better to have loved and lived than to have watched on the sidelines waiting for your turn to play.

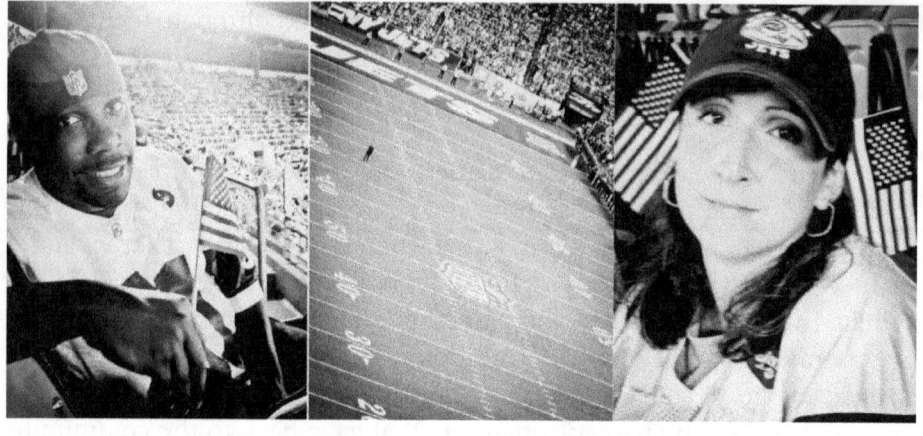

I can walk away from a fight and know the difference between insecurity and fear. The skill sets that I learned have helped me run a school, a photography business and to be an effective life-coach. I actually have to separate myself from the term life-coach because I do more than that. As the LifeSensei I believe I have to answer only to GOD in heaven; my goal is to be a voice for those that can't be heard. To be an imperfect example to those that may think like me or feel like me. There is a difference between cockiness and confidence. I am confident. "My desire" has always been to know my role in life and be comfortable with it. Now that I know who I am, it is easier for me to help others discover themselves.

As a New Yorker, I can be emotionally cold sometimes, a product of a city that forced me to harden in order to survive. I was raised by my family to be independent; I didn't realize that meant being alone. **Independent is defined as: a (1) : not subject to control by others : self-governing (2) : not affiliated with a larger controlling unit b (1) : not requiring or relying on something else : not contingent 2) : not looking to others for one's opinions or for guidance in conduct (3) : not bound by or committed to a political party c (1) : not requiring or relying on others (as for care or livelihood)d : showing a desire for freedom** I was taught me to be independent and responsible before adding additional responsibilities. Life is complicated enough; please do not make life worse for yourself. Whether you like it or not life is going to be difficult.

I guess my passion for life told me this was the way to go. I am stubbornly old-school, some say an old soul. This isn't just about my dreams; this is about yours too, whatever they may be, whatever you may decide to do in life, whatever you might want to accomplish. I hope that this book finds you in reasonable health and full of hope and dreams. I pray that this does sound a little corny to you and touches your heart. If I sound sarcastic or harsh sometimes it is because I am, but my advice and views are well-intentioned. As a Martial Arts instructor and fitness trainer, I have found that the simple, straight forward approach works best for me. My wish for you is success; not just with finding motivation, or getting in shape. My wish for you is to be successful in all aspects of life and to have an abundant life. This is possible whether you are black or white, short or tall, single or married, alone or wanting to be alone.

This book is an ode to the average person doing above average things, great things. Will you join me in celebrating you? This book is dedicated to anyone who picked up a weight, jogged, swam, tried out for a team or wanted not to be picked last. This is dedicated to everyone who wished they were someone else, and to those who had the courage to be unique. This is for all of you who do not look at scales, eat what you want or watch what you eat.

This is for the late night binger and for those who purge themselves after a meal. This is for the bullies and those that are bullied, for the street conscious and the unaware. This is for those who want answers but do not know who to ask or where to look. This is for parents who give up and for those who try too hard, for the teen who is searching, or the adult who knows everything.

This is for the radicals, skeptics, and critics who want to tell you what you can and cannot do. This is for those that want and believe there is something more out there and are willing to go get it.

This is for you!

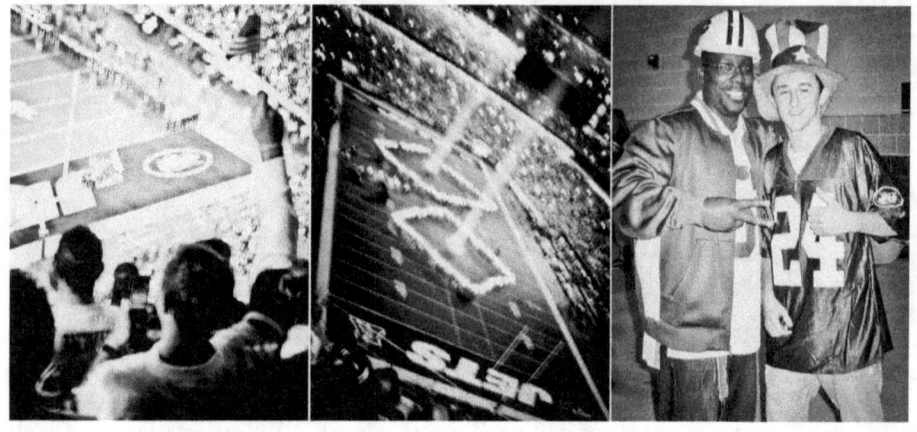

The Trained mentality prepares you to see and do things a little differently. The Trained concept is loosely based on the subway system. It's real, direct, and purposeful, whatever your goal or destination. The idea of being trained is to do what doesn't come to you naturally, through hard work and discipline, to see results from your labor that will benefit you and others for years to come; to revel in your accomplishments because you dared to set them and you prevailed.

That is just the New Yorker in me, we are more than conquerors. Having the benefit of meeting people in life who saved, gave and paved the way for me; I hope I can honor them by helping you. The Trained mindset can and will help get you where you want or need to be. I can't sleep if I'm not being real. Being real to me means giving back and watching each other's back.

We see results doing things the right way. Simple, proven methods cultivated and acquired by experience and sharing positive values. While many take shortcuts, the easy way out only guarantees one thing. Not being consistently successful. At some point, one way or another they are going to need to be trained the right way. That's where I come in.

Let's get you in the best shape possible-mentally, spiritually, emotionally and, of course, physically. When done correctly, it not only feels right, you know you look good inside and out. That is and should always be the goal, whether you start today or tomorrow. Regardless of your perceived shortcomings, setbacks and obstacles, taking the steps to read this book will ensure you a better future.

You are not alone out there. This book and this journey are to be shared.

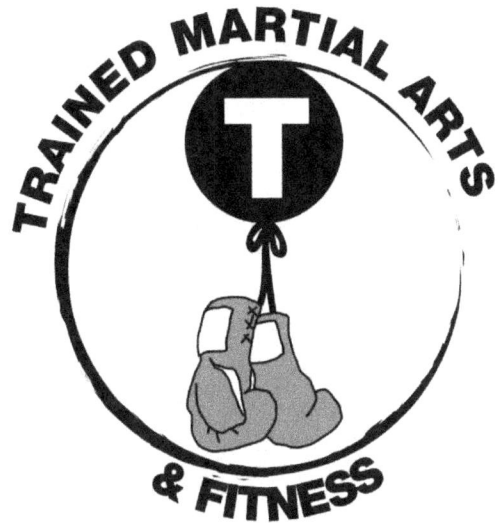

As always,

Live, Love and Laugh

Terence Mitchell

The Life Sensei on Fitness Crazes

Why you keep changing your workout

For many people, trying out different workouts, classes, gyms and diets is a way to break up boring patterns and add variety to their workout routines.

The problem begins when you spend more time looking for the next big trend and notice consistently smaller results. Results seem great in the beginning but trail off when your focus wanes.

Your body and mind craves variety but at some point the fitness crazes just ends up making you crazy.

Martial Arts, Yoga, Gymnastics, and Dance are the core disciplines that will consistently benefit you the most. They force you to focus and develop a skill set.

That's why instructors keep on changing their classes to fit society's need for the next big thing, while emptying your wallet in the process. They also distract you from focusing on long term results.

Think about it; boxing, aero-boxing, cardio boxing, dance boxing, kickboxing (fitness), they are all taking the elements of boxing and diluting the true benefits to make you feel more comfortable.

In the process, you are developing habits that are contrary to actually boxing. So if the music, instructor, time slot, and classmates change so do you.

What skill set did you acquire and positive habits did you form?

The same can be said of Pilates, Dance classes, Weight training Yoga, etc. Keep it simple, keep on going to class, and learn something.

Develop a new skill set, and build positive habits avoid craziness.

Martial guidance for life's journey

The economy may be tough but air is still free

Proper breathing technique is extremely important during training. Breathing supplies oxygen to the muscle cells, which is essential for muscle contraction, and helps deliver energy and build the muscle. Make sure to exhale when you lift the weight and inhale when you lower it.

Remember to breathe properly when doing any exercise.

Rest - Take a break from exercise or any type of movement that may stress the injured area. A minor injury should be rested for one or two days, while more severe injuries may need longer.

Ice - Ice the affected area. Icing reduces pain, limits swelling and bleeding, and encourages rapid healing. Wrap ice in a towel to avoid direct contact with the skin.

Compress - Compress the injury with a stretch bandage. Make sure not to wrap it too tight, just enough to support the injured area comfortably.

Elevate - Elevate the limb. If possible, try to keep the injured part above the level of the heart. At the very least, try to keep it higher than the hips. This helps limit swelling and also prevents movement of the area that is injured.

Beginner Arms

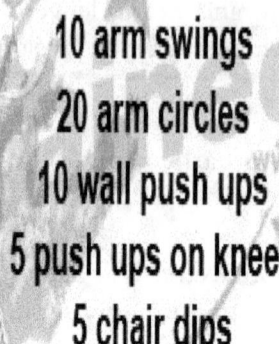

10 arm swings
20 arm circles
10 wall push ups
5 push ups on knees
5 chair dips
2 squat thrusts
:10 sec plank
10 wall push ups
5 chair dips
30 weightless bicep curls
10 arm swings
:30 tricep stretch each arm

theLifeSenSei.trainerze.com for the videos to exercises

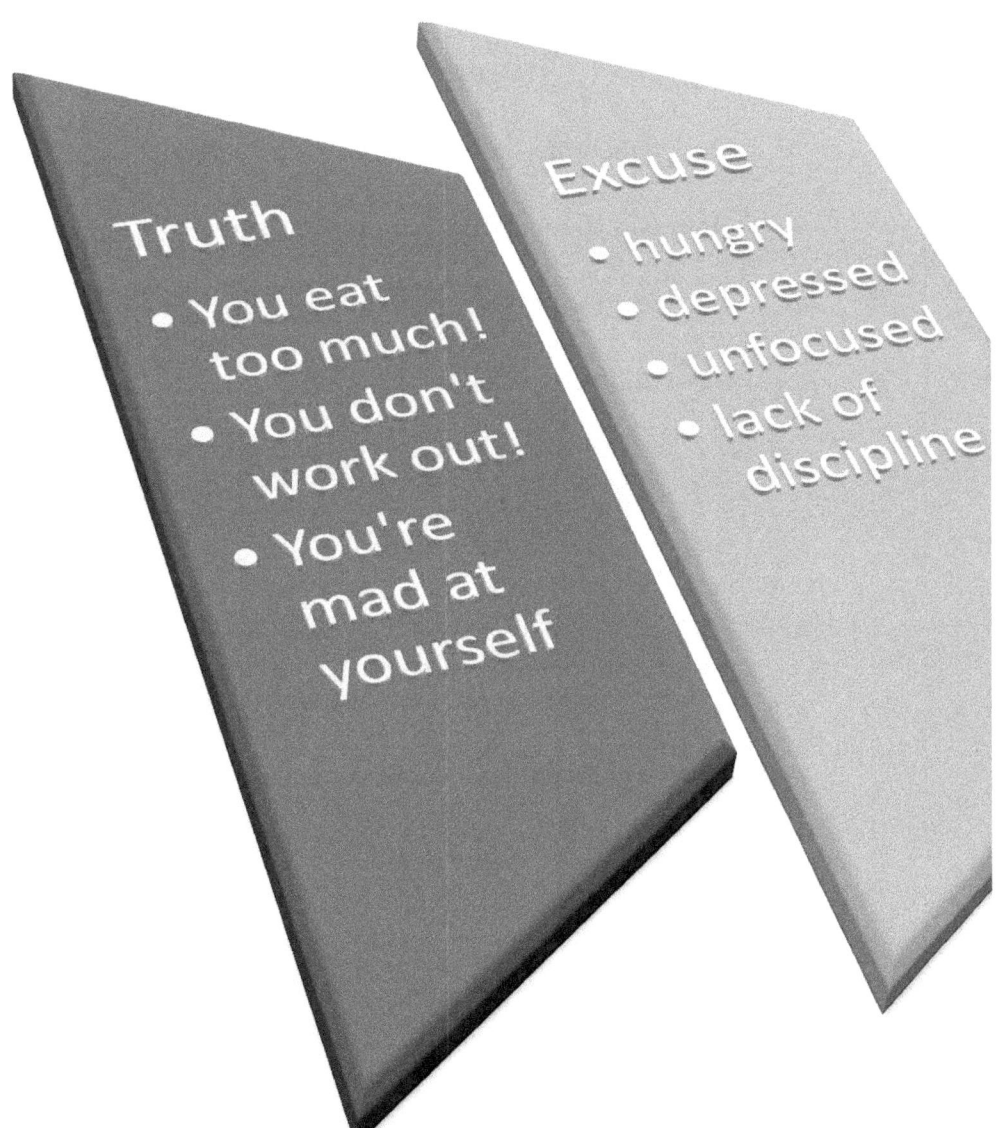

Plan

Many people think that working out to lose weight is too much work

Almost everyone believes they are going to put the weight back

Success comes with proper guidance and the right attitude

Implement

Change the way you think about losing weight

Invest in yourself with time, money, energy

Invest in your body with healthy choices

Invest until you see results

Habit

Stress relief

Hit an inanimate object till you can't anymore, e.g. Heavy bag

Talk to a good active listener

Go outside get some fresh air breath inhale +exhale

Result

Jumping Jacks

Traditional, military, Squat Jacks

Change the tempo, pause + hold position, work up to 5-10 min

1st *Stop:* *How to be Successful When Training*

One of the most frequent questions asked regarding getting in shape, is, "will I be able to accomplish this?" Will I ever get fit? The answer is yes! Every time I hear that question I'm amazed because most people cannot see themselves doing things that are successive, different, and/or challenging. Somewhere we've forgotten how to explore new things, expand our knowledge base and honestly, be more physical. This has become more apparent, more problematic for our society, endangering our lives socially, mentally, emotionally and physically.

As our world continues to lose more of its natural habitat, with our parks, hiking trails, and national treasures making way for condos, strip malls and real estate ventures, we find ourselves staying at home more. The criminal element has made it almost impossible to leave our children out on the street to play stickball or basketball. We allow our kids to become increasingly physically inactive. We grow more in love with our entertainment systems, video games, tablets and the almighty bed. The average home now spends seven hours of the day watching TV. Although statistics, reality TV and the media all point to it, the American population is considering if it is actually obese or unfit.

We use to work out when we were younger, when it required little effort. We use to work out when our parents took us to afterschool programs, when our best friends forced us to go. We worked out when we saw immediate results and we were not so busy, and when we use to play on teams and our bodies naturally kept its shape.

I've been there too. I've thought about staying home versus working out. I go to the movies and want a tub of popcorn and soda. I like a nice meal at a fancy restaurant and some delicious dessert. I notice the younger people and realize I'm getting older. That is where it ends though; I cannot afford to stop training. It is not only my livelihood, but it makes me feel whole inside.

I have to take advantage of time and make the most out of the day. That means working on something to further my goals, so I can find success in my endeavors. Just like everyone else, I take breaks, skip a workout or two. I get overwhelmed with work, even when work is training people. Sometimes I do not want to put on the gloves to box, or stretch before doing jiu-jitsu. It is easier to watch for proper technique, than it is, to work out with the personal training clients. Life happens, we get sick, want to rest, have a drink, be lazy. We want to hang with friends, be entertained, and focus on loved ones. We want to eat what we want, live how we want and working out is just not a priority.

So here we all are at home, wishing we got out more. We blame it on the kids, and our significant others. We get out of the house to go to work, drop the kids off, or to get away from the craziness once in a while. We run our errands on the weekend or when we have free time, often not being able to tell the difference between running errands and free time. We sometimes go out to the movies, or watch sports games, go to clubs, bars or parties. We often go out to eat fast food, a late night meal or for dessert. We do all these things without a second thought, closing our eyes as we settle into a comfortable position into bed as we fall asleep. We can all agree that we all feel tired.

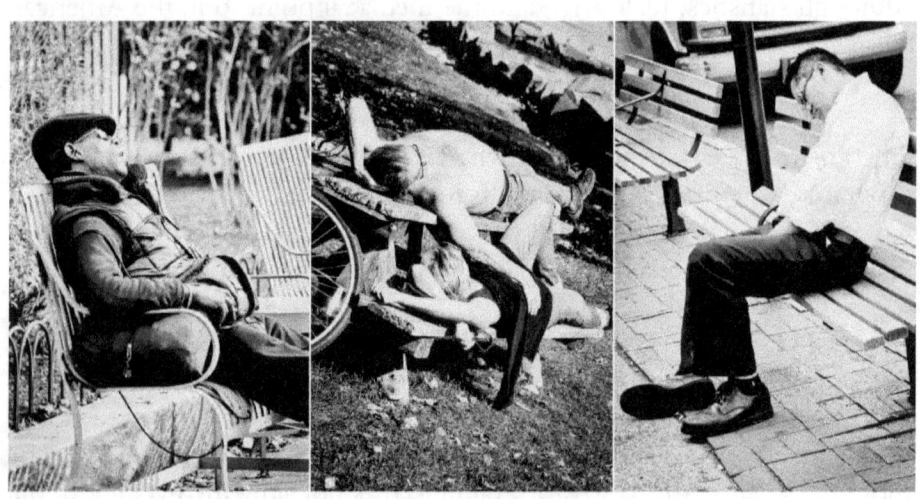

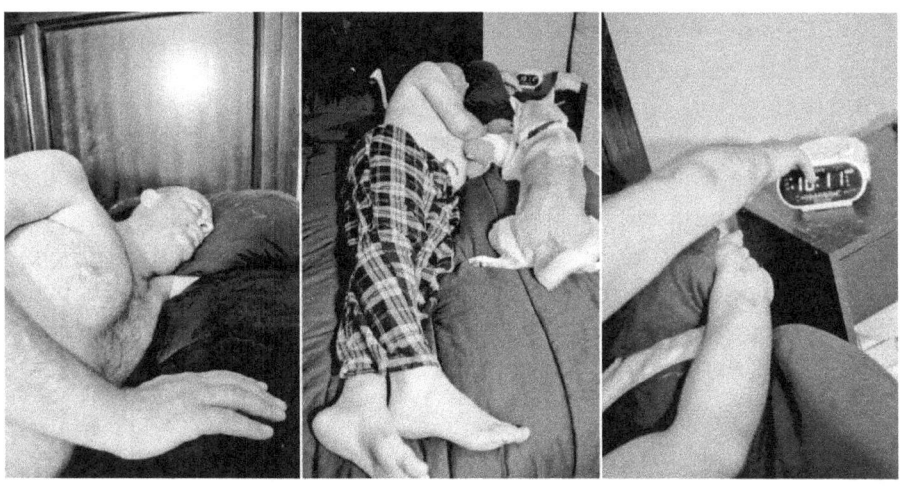

Wake Up! Stay with me as I guess your morning routine. You wake up feeling heavy and unattractive. Staring at the mirror naked, you look at the closet with disgust. Your stomach rumbles, begging for something healthy inside, reminding you of that upcoming event this weekend. Getting on the scale you step off, stand a little straighter and repeat the process. Sometimes, you get up rub your belly and shake your head. Thinking it is time to make a change, you secretly swear off that dessert you swallowed whole last night. It must be a magic mirror that you continue to stare at, waiting for your dream body to pop into view. Looking for that belt with the extra loop you struggle to conceal your gut, or you look for another pair of pants as you tuck in your shirt and rush to work.

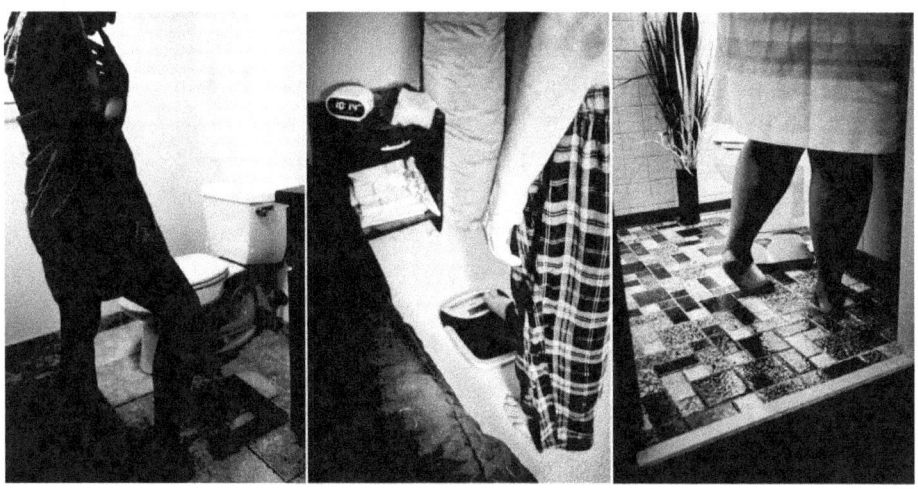

Parents, you comment on how you wish your child was more active and try to remember what you did as a child to stay in shape. You think about getting in shape, but how? There is no time; your job has begun to define who you are, between the commute, short lunch and responsibilities it is not feasible to believe you can consistently train so, why bother? The barbecue is next weekend, so you can start after that. No one looks like those models on TV, so it is not a big deal. Buying clothes that fit you better is easier. As you leave your house you see someone jogging, and you wish you had that type of motivation. Drinking your coffee gets you pumped, you decide you are going to find a gym to get fit.

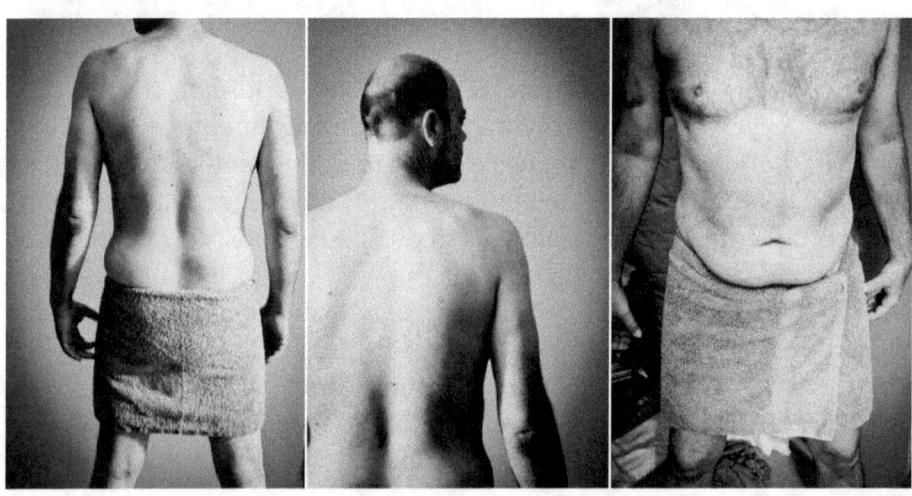

You get excited as you begin to think about how life would be better if you had a new body. As the day continues, you think about what you would wear. You think about activities you would enjoy, things you would do with your family in your new fit body. You would live differently, eat healthier, be happier and life would be awesome! It does not matter how much you lose, if you just lost ten pounds it would be the start that would change everything. You eat at a healthy restaurant for lunch and think you might throw up. You talk to your co-workers about your ideas and they smile to your face but laugh when you walk away. You notice how that guy/girll seems to have a lovely physique, they work out and seem happy. When you look online under fitness and see tons of different gyms, you roll your eyes in frustration and continue on with your day.

Sound familiar? You are obviously not alone. Unfortunately, we all end the evening the same way, forgetting how we felt in the morning. We pass the gyms, fitness centers, bike pathways, and jogging trails. We skip the home gym, and walk past the fitness DVD's and lay our clothing on our treadmills. Devouring whatever we want, we slouch on the couch watching our favorite TV shows, eating on our sizeable portion plates. We ponder our existence after our second or third helping of food. Then we're off to the freezer for an extra scoop of ice cream to compensate for our guilt. Why get out of bed and stare in the mirror when you know what you looked like the night before? Here is an opportunity to get in shape. Get out of bed and do five, ten, or twenty pushups and sit ups instead. Rather than stepping on the scale, throw on some shorts and run up and down a flight of steps twenty times or for five to ten minutes. Take the clothes off the treadmill or home gym and exercise for thirty minutes and then start your day. If you were to do this for one month you would begin to see a difference. What are you waiting for? Every day starts with a game plan, big or small. Change your life today.

Visualize & Actualize

You look at yourself first thing in the morning because you want to see what everyone else will see first. That is how we all judge one another. Many people say we'd rather be with someone who makes us laugh over good looks, meaning we want substance more than the visual. Is this actually true? Wouldn't you rather have both? Your boss gives the employee who stands straighter the raise. The more athletic child gets the start in games. The more physically fit you are, the more opportunities you have. Need benefits for exercise? Working out will lead to increased lean body mass and less fat. It will lower your blood pressure and improve your outlook on life. The benefits to working out are without end. All over the internet, in books and conversations, the common sense wisdom says: The more you work out, the more likely you will be successful.

"I exercised once, but found I was allergic to it. My skin flushed and my heart raced. I got sweaty and short of breath. Very dangerous" – Anonymous

Success in training starts with a mindset. **Mindset is defined as a set of beliefs or a way of thinking that determines somebody's behavior and outlook.** The truth is that we all have to start somewhere. I can remember the first time I took a karate class, how awkward I felt being in a uniform. Everyone was watching me or so I thought. I also remember the feeling of a job well done after my first karate class, the feeling of accomplishment that I earned, after doing something I didn't think I could do. The first time I rollerbladed in NYC, I was happy to have on my safety gear after the thirtieth fall. I remember thinking that one day I would be able to rollerblade throughout the city without falling.

The successful mindset does not leave room for second-guessing, inactivity, laziness, the word "tomorrow" or the phrase "next year." The successful mindset doesn't "envy", it "**admires**", and it doesn't "want" it "**needs.**" It doesn't "wish" it "**makes happen.**" The successful mindset knows that each day promises new adventures instead of challenges, new goals instead of setbacks.

Procrastinating

Everyone has fears. *Fear* **is defined as to be afraid of: expect with alarm.** I was afraid of rollerblading and falling down on the hard concrete pavement while honking cars swerved out of the way. But, by the time the sun went down, I rollerbladed for more than fifty blocks. Sure some people laughed when I fell down, but that's their problem, because I was rollerblading and they were walking. Did I think after my first karate lesson I'd inherit Bruce Lee's spirit and become an overnight success? I hated looking in the mirror throwing the wrong technique, or watching myself huff and puff trying to catch my breath while everyone else appeared to be in great shape. I failed to notice as I was watching everyone else, that no one was paying attention to me, everyone was more concerned with themselves.

The Life Sensei says, "Think about it"

How you approach problems usually dictates how you will deal with them.

My fear and worrying did not get me anywhere, and I was missing out on the finer points of class. I went home and I was sore for a few days after the first week karate ended. I thought my instructor was a nut job. Yet I was one week closer to black belt.

Let's rewind for a bit and go back in time. Let's say I never took that karate class, I might not have developed the confidence to get out of retail. I would not have become a personal trainer and would not have earned the title of Sensei. The opportunity to become a business owner would not have come up. I would not have been able to work for myself for over twelve years. I would not have had the opportunity to change lives through life coaching and help others reach their goals. Most importantly you would not be reading this book. A lot of people see the benefits of karate (loosely translated as "empty hand training"), but do not think it is for them. The uniforms, screaming, bowing to one another and getting hit do not seem to be worth the hassle. The feeling of accomplishment after receiving a belt, learning to control your emotions and temperament, having respect for yourself and others, learning how to take punishment and dish it out if warranted is something everyone should experience. Developing discipline, finding out what you're capable of, setting challenges and completing them that is building a fear-proof foundation.

Many people wear uniforms to work including suits and dresses. We scream at each other from our homes to the road and to our offices. We are taught to respect others at an early age and generally show our elders, peers, and those in authority. We fight mentally, verbally and physically and often without effort and rarely with skill. The outcome is often the same…pointless. So why is martial art training so feared?

I made a decision to stop worrying about things I could not change; I was tired of living in a self-made prison of the mind. Worrying gets you nowhere and your worries become your reality if you let them. Karate for me was the spark that got me into Krav Maga, Jiu-Jitsu, Kickboxing and Boxing to name a few. It made me one of the few African-American business owners in my area and allowed me to live my dreams. That was some karate class huh?

My game plan was simple; I didn't want to be afraid anymore. Not afraid of success, of failure, of others and most importantly of myself. Karate was a means to not being afraid; roller blades were a means of cheap transport (I hate to drive) and most New Yorkers will tell you they hate to drive too. So I bought a pair of overly priced rollerblades and **committed** to busting my butt every three blocks.

The Life Sensei says, "Think about it"

To be successful you have to start, that's it. Not tomorrow not in fifteen minutes. Right Now!

Again, Karate worked for me; you might need a different spark. There are plenty of them out there, do something new and exciting. Instead of worrying about the results just go out and have some fun. Discover a new hobby, a new passion and be successful at it.

The Life Sensei's quick tips

Be realistic with your game plan, start out slowly. If you do start right now, you are already closer to your goals than you were before. Here are a few tips:

1. **Be conscious of time.**

2. **Set realistic goals.**

3. **Plan variety to prevent laziness and boredom from setting in.**

4. **Start slower than your initial game plan.**

5. **You want to train smarter not harder so that you can make this a life style change and not a life threatening one.**

Now go see a doctor to make sure you can start training.

Trained 2 B Tips:

Stick with your resolutions

- Focus on positive self-talk. Congratulate yourself every time you take a step towards your resolution goal. Be your own best cheerleader.
- Avoid berating yourself if you should fall back or break a resolution. Just brush yourself off and start over again.
- Stick to your resolution by considering it a promise to yourself, not a test of your willpower.
- Avoid situations that put you in temptation's path, meaning if you're on a diet, do not go to the ice cream parlor.
- Keep a sticky note in a prominent place so that you see it every day, reminding yourself of your resolutions. (On your bathroom mirror, next to your bed, on the refrigerator)
- Be realistic. Make sure your plan is a realistic one that can fit into your lifestyle. Will you really have the energy to go out for that evening exercise class? Make changes as easy and convenient as possible.

TRUTH

No one said that getting started will be easy, what are you waiting for? Your goals are attainable, but you have to really want to see change. Learn to accept your body and work to make yourself comfortable in your body. One step at a time with a solid desire to get in shape, solid plan and solid mindset will produce solid results.

Get rid of flabby arms

10 pushups

24 bicep burners

15 shoulder presses

10 diamond pushups

15 tricep dips

15 bent over rows

15 lateral raises

10 wide grip push ups

15 tricep kickbacks

1000 punches or

500 on a heavy bag

theLifeSenSei.trainerze.com for the videos to exercises

The Life Sensei on Weights

Weight Training Basics You Need to Know

Common exercise recommendation is for three sets of ten repetitions of an exercise (3x10) ex. three sets of ten squats.

Try lighter or heavier weights for comfort with useful intensity. You should rest between sets so that your body replenishes its energy system for the next round.

Tempo is the speed at which you lift the weight. You should vary the tempo at which you train, by changing the tempo you will increase the time under tension and force the muscles to adapt.

When designing a program make sure that the program trains both the pushing and pulling muscle groups. This prevents imbalances and the potential for self induced injuries from improper training!

I focus all my clients on real world strength or functional strength. By training the grip you will have more wrist control (less injury) and also you will be able to focus more and that will allow you to recruit more muscle fibers thus making you stronger. Do not bend your wrists.

Don't over train. Get a trainer, instructor, or coach if you want to take yourself to the next level, until you feel comfortable enough to train on your own.

Hyperextension means pushing a joint beyond its normal range of movement. This may produce injury when excessive joint movement stresses ligaments and tendons. A slight flex of the joint is all that is required to prevent the possible hyperextension.

Switch your work out times; everyone has different energy levels throughout the day. This will challenge you even if you're using the same weights.

Home Workout Basic

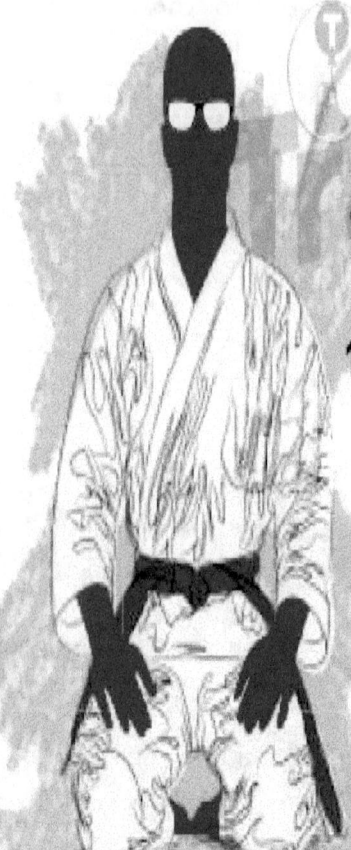

10 high knees
10 jumping jacks
10 lying leg raises
10 push ups
10 lunges each leg
10 bicycles
:10 sec plank
:10 wall squat
10 A squats
10 squat thrusts

theLifeSenSei.trainerze.com for the videos to exercises

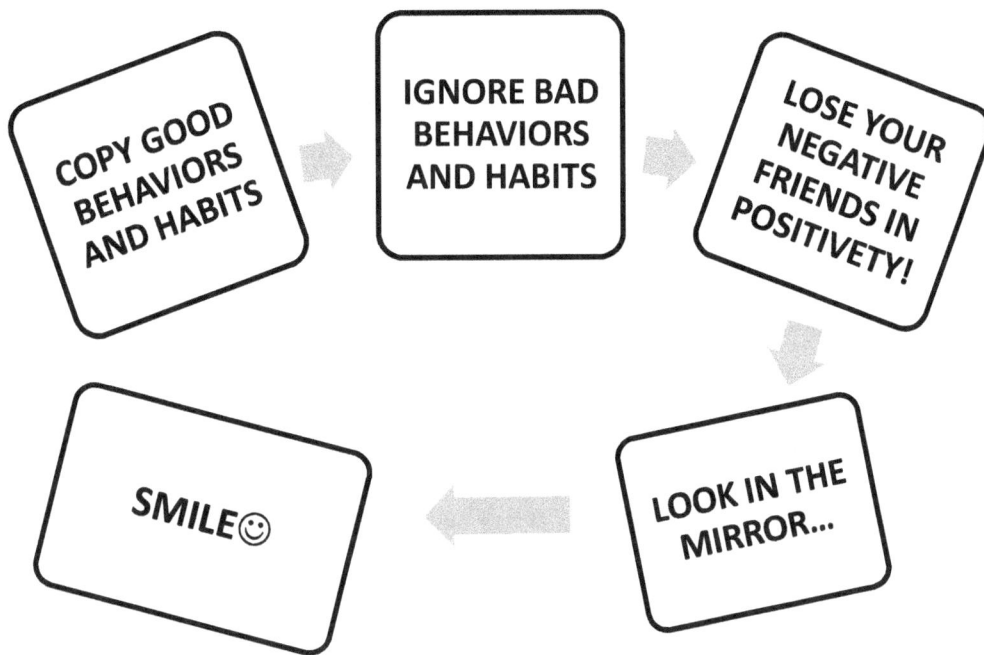

The Life Sensei says, "Think about it"

Everybody has to start somewhere. For you, now is when! Mentally, the hardest part is you wanting something more for yourself. Let go of fears. Dream big! Want more. Go for it. Visualize success and begin to make it happen.

SIMPLE: Wait for the book to magically transform you.

AVERAGE: Put off tomorrow what you can do today.

GREAT! : Think about where you see yourself being in five months and plan accordingly.

BALANCE: Find thirty minutes in your day to be healthier. That is four and a half hrs a week, eighteen hours a month, you get the idea.

The Life Sensei "Your body reflects your habits"

What your body really says about you

It doesn't matter how big or small you appear to be, if you are disabled or suffering from an injury your body will tell a story about you.

We have learned to build defenses around these stories because we are uncomfortable with how honest our bodies are.

I am in the possession of skinny legs, a protruding stomach and poor eyesight. I can't change that, it's a part of me. When I don't work out consistently, the first thing you will notice is how skinny my legs are, and that my stomach protrudes. That is one story. What characteristics define your body?

Having said that I work out to be comfortable and healthy; finding a balance with my body while paying special attention to my legs, and abdominals. That is another story. What story does your body tell?

Our body stores excess fat when our eating habits aren't trustworthy, when we choose to avoid exercise and our metabolism slows down. Our body then loses muscle tone, while our cardiovascular abilities and our desire to be energetic weaken as a result. This is a fairly common story, yet we are still so defensive about it. There is no reason to be defensive any longer.

We live in a world now when anyone regardless of physical capability can find an activity that will tell a story about their body that they can be comfortable with. Let your body reflect good habits.

What defenses have you built due to your discomfort?

Are your habits beneficial or detrimental to your health?

The story is up to you, make it an interesting one.

Martial guidance for life's journey

Check your heart rate

Unless you are working out within your target heart rate range, you are not reaping the cardiovascular and fat burning benefits of the exercise. To find your target heart rate, subtract your age from 220 (this is your maximum heart rate). It is recommended that you work out at about 70% of your target heart rate zone when starting out. So, if you're 30 years old, your maximum heart rate would be 190 beats per minute and working out at 70% of that would put your heart rate at about 133 beats per minute (190 multiplied by 0.7). As your level of fitness improves, you can up that number to 161 beats per minute. A quick way of calculating your target heart rate during exercise is to take your pulse for 10 seconds and multiply the number of beats by 6.

Love your Legs

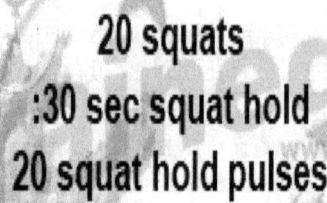

20 squats
:30 sec squat hold
20 squat hold pulses

20 alternating lunge kicks
20 jump lunges
:30 sec lunge hold each side

20 calf raises
20 more toes in
20 more toes out
repeat total set 3 x

theLifeSenSei.trainerze.com for the videos to exercises

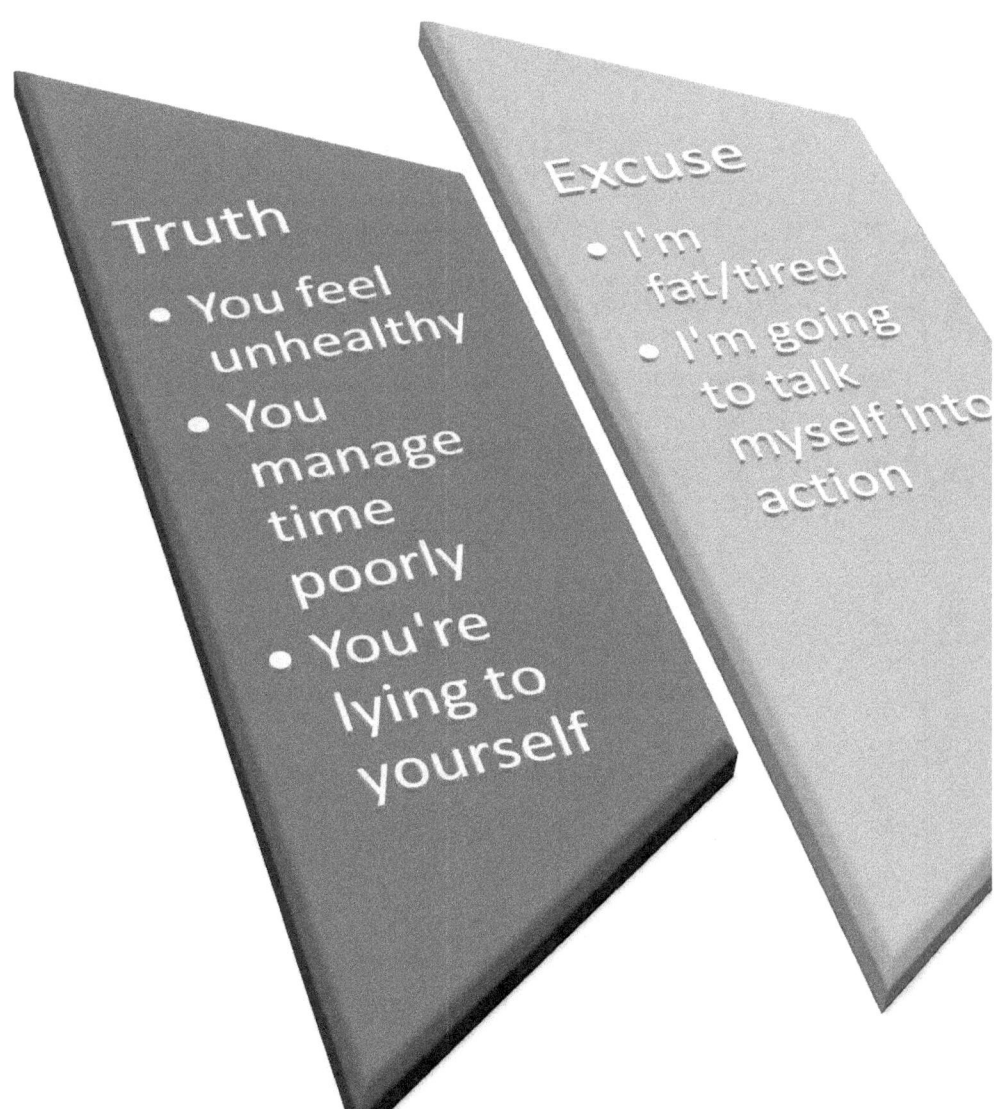

Truth
- You feel unhealthy
- You manage time poorly
- You're lying to yourself

Excuse
- I'm fat/tired
- I'm going to talk myself into action

Plan

More sleep = better choices

Choices + results = more successful you

Success + recovery time = value every second daily

Make every second count + doing your best = time to sleep

Implement

Work in intervals

Give Me 3 sets and 6 to 10 reps of whatever you do

6 reps for heavy weights 8 reps for resistance training 10 reps for cardio

If 3 sets are easy increase sets/ decrease time to complete

Habit

Building Confidence

Think of the Happiest Moment in your Life

Make a list of only your top 20 favorite songs

Think about a moment when you were truly successful

Result

Lunges: Total lower body workout

Traditional, Crossing, Reverse, Jump

For tight butt, toned thighs, balance and strength

2nd *Stop: Realistic Fitness Goals*

Think about how often you wanted to get in shape. What prevented you? If you could see how being in shape is vital and no longer optional, you would be motivated to do something about it. What are the benefits to being healthy? Seeing the world, as opposed to watching it on your TV, living a longer life, avoiding time in the hospital, spending more time with your family, being productive, working on making more babies, seeing your great grandkids first play.

Why do you want to be fit? Visually, if you are fit you could be seen as sexy, desirable and athletic. These are all associated with working out. Need a boost to be successful financially? It helps being fit. Want to get that job, promotion, raise, business deal? Do you want to be seen as determined, intelligent, hardworking, passionate, and strong-willed? All these traits are associated with being fit. Looking for that special someone? What ad would catch your eye?

OBESE, LAZY, COUCH POTATO NOT CONCERNED WITH APPEARANCE. LOOKING FOR AN OUT-OF-SHAPE,

INACTIVE SLEEP SPECIALIST LONGING FOR NAPS,

FAST FOOD MEALS AND RE RUNS OF SHOWS ON CABLE NETWORKS.

Sound like a dream date to you? Me neither. Let's get started. Grab a jump rope and start jumping, put on your running sneakers and start jogging. Go to the nearest gym and start lifting weights. Feel the excitement of running on the treadmill or working the elliptical again. If you think it's that simple you are wrong. If you do not believe me, get some healthy popcorn and go to your nearest gym. Find a spot where you won't get in anyone's way and watch. You can't just jump into a routine or program. You have to be educated and prepared. Start jumping without stretching and you can get a calf or ankle injury. Now you have to wait till you get healed. Start running without a game plan or proper running techniques and you can get shin splints; knee injuries or worse suffer from sheer boredom and hang up your sneakers for good.

Having a realistic fitness goal is more than just being physical. This is a key point to the trained mentality. You need to have several things working in your favor: An understanding of why, realizing every little bit counts, simple steps to improve your workout and building consistency.

Wow, that seems like a lot of work when you think about it. It's no wonder most people do not work out effectively. They factor in not having enough time, or money. When in truth what they do not have is **resolve**. So, let's get some firmness (in our minds, hearts and buttocks).

Remember your childhood dreams of being an American superstar, professional athlete, stunt driver, or celebrity? Now think back and try to remember if any of your childhood idols were out of shape. Did you say as a child I want to be an out of shape star? Did you want to look and feel unhealthy? Think about today's celebrities that may be considered overweight. Think about how often they are asked about their weight, go on public diets, and gain the weight back only to diet again. Think about how Jessica is glamorized when she is thin and vilified when she puts on some weight. The same people who point out how great she looked in those daisy dukes now make fun of her for being an overweight country star. I want you to think about where you are now. It is never too late to get in shape or reach your childhood dreams.

The Life Sensei says, "Think about it"

Getting into shape is no longer optional; working out is a necessity.

Understanding why you work out is crucial for you to remain consistent with your workout. When you feel like you cannot continue, you will want to remember why you are working out. Now I am not talking about weddings, vacations, first dates, new jobs etc. Most people are motivated enough to get in shape for an event and equally motivated to quit after it is over.

Those reasons are temporary; you cannot hold on to the focus you have when it is just for a specific occasion. The results are temporary also, ensuring you will repeat the same mistakes. What we are talking about here is life style change. Why are high school and college reunions so popular? Everyone wants to see what has become of each other. Did the high school sport star marry the prom queen? Did the resident genius make it big? And let's not forget the proverbial "ugly duckling"; heads turn, tongues drop as that relative unknown "average person" becomes the bombshell or stud that everyone dreams about. Similarly, I would be a millionaire if I had a dollar for every person that wanted to get in shape in one month to go on vacation. The usual mindset is they are going to quit eating, workout harder than they ever did before and lose all the weight they put on for years in one month. In this miracle month all of the unhealthy habits they formed will be broken. They will scour the internet for dieting tips. They will sell part of their soul to fit in a special outfit so their vacation will be considered a success. **That type of thinking sets us up to fail because it is shortsighted.**

If we were to workout, get in shape, maintain our fitness level at an above average level, for the duration of each year we would live a less stressful life. You would spend less time visiting doctors, or seeing a pharmacist. You would be confident when going on that first date or boardroom meeting. You would enjoy engaging in physical activities rather than worrying about your appearance, breathing capabilities, and wondering if you are in proper shape. We would not have to freak out before significant engagements, family functions, vacations in warm weather or accidentally bumping in to our exes. **Understanding why is to prevent injury, maintain healthiness and develop peace of mind.**

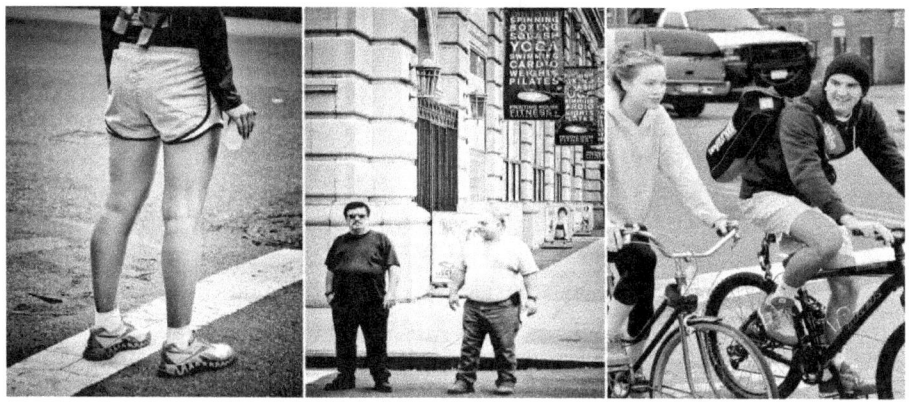

REALIZING EVERY LITTLE BIT COUNTS

You do not start training for a marathon by running a marathon. You start by running a little bit here and a little bit there. Beginning with a successful mindset follows with starting, going one step at a time and continues with sticking to a routine. Was Rome built in a day? Neither was the Great Wall of China, or the Apple dynasty. Day by day, add something new to the way you train. Give yourself a chance to make it a habit by taking baby steps. When it becomes part of your daily regimen, duplicate it.

For example; this may start with going to bed at a reasonable time, and setting your alarm. Set it loud enough so that you get up on time. Set your clock at least five minutes earlier and stretch, eventually fifteen minutes then thirty. Before you know it you're getting up earlier and doing a light routine. Your metabolism gets an earlier start than you're used to plus you can burn fat throughout the day. Your confidence improves gradually as you reinforce positive behaviors. Now you are ready to take the next step.

The Life Sensei says, "Think about it"

Find a trainer and/or a workout partner. What you should look for is someone who doesn't take themselves too seriously, but is serious about getting you in shape, same goes for your partner.

Find a gym where you can speak to someone who will personally help you reach your goals. Find someone who is knowledgeable and willing to help make you look and feel good. If your personal trainer asks you to do something, you should feel comfortable doing it. Certificates help, but understand that there are many wacky people with them as well. Contrary to popular belief, there is no universal governing body on fitness, so do not believe the hype. Many businesses use certificates as a form of insurance. If you are willing to put your health in the hands of someone who got their certificate on "low cost personal training certification dot com", be my guest. Experience is the best teacher. Just because your trainer has rock hard abs or a tight backside doesn't mean they know how to help you see the same results.

A certificate won't tell you if they really know what they are talking about, have experience helping others or are successful at what they do. Ask to watch them train someone with needs similar to yours. **You are in business, the business of investing in yourself to get in the shape that will help you be the most successful.** Do not allow your dreams to be ruined before they start with a personal trainer or instructor from Hell. Next, find a training buddy. We have all heard this before. If your training partner doesn't like the same type of workouts that you do, find one who will hold you accountable, who can tell you to get off your lazy rump and won't offend you too badly. Find someone who can give you constructive advice. Find someone who you look up to who also looks up to you, someone who you can set achievable goals together.

Good ideas for training partners:

Family members (not to far apart in age)

Significant others (make sure goals are the same)

Coworkers (leave work then work out)

Pets (will listen and out run you)

Best friends (you owe them and they owe you)

Teammates (set your sights on team unity)

Write out your goals with your partner. No really write them out. It's proven when you write something and/or read it you will retain it longer. Figure out a timetable of when you want to achieve your goals. Write out a realistic schedule of when you are going to train. Also, write out an alternative plan in case you miss a workout, as well as a punishment for skipping a workout altogether. In case of inclement weather, plan potential options for indoor workouts. Plan for outdoor activities when your school or gym is closed to prevent missing workouts. Have the mind set to be one step ahead of your evil, lazy, unmotivated alter ego. Be sure to use a workout log to record your progress and be sure to communicate openly with your partner.

NO EXCUSES

THINGS TO AVOID IN YOUR

WORKOUT ROUTINE

WAKE UP LATE

STARE AT THE MIRROR

DO NOT WORKOUT

DISTRACTING OTHERS FROM THEIR WORKOUT

TALKING TOO MUCH & DOING TOO LITTLE

CALL YOUR TRAINING PARTNER AND TELL THEM YOU CAN'T MAKE IT

GET TO YOUR SESSION OR CLASS LATE

MAKE EXCUSES

WORKING OUT AND NOT PUSHING YOURSELF

DO NOT STRETCH BEFORE OR AFTER YOU WORKOUT

DO NOT DRINK ENOUGH WATER

Try your best not to be cheap with your workouts. You weren't cheap when you were adding that extra scoop of cookie dough ice cream in you bowl. When you order the large soda and popcorn combo in the movie theatre, you weren't cutting corners either. The only person you hurt when you slack from your routine is yourself. Push yourself a little bit harder each time. Encourage one another often and do not be cheap about that either. Everyone needs encouragement.

SIMPLE STEPS TO IMPROVE YOUR WORKOUT

GET SEVEN TO EIGHT HOURS OF SLEEP

WAKE UP EARLY

WORKOUT-BE CONSISTENT

STRETCH/DRINK WATER

EAT BREAKFAST

EAT A SNACK

STRETCH/DRINK WATER

WORKOUT-TRAIN DIFFERENT MUSCLES

EAT LUNCH

EAT A SNACK

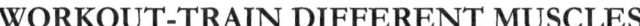

WORKOUT-DO SOMETHING FUN!

EAT DINNER

STRETCH/DRINK WATER

GO TO BED AT A REASONABLE TIME

Find variations that work for you. Look at that list again. What is the one thing that is repeated the most? Yep, read it and weep stretching; otherwise known as the anti-workout. One of the simplest ways to improve health is to stretch. That doesn't necessarily mean yoga, although that is a possible supplement. What it does mean is along with cardio, weight lifting, building core strength; you should definitely stretch as often as you can. Make time to stretch before you work out or after you are done.

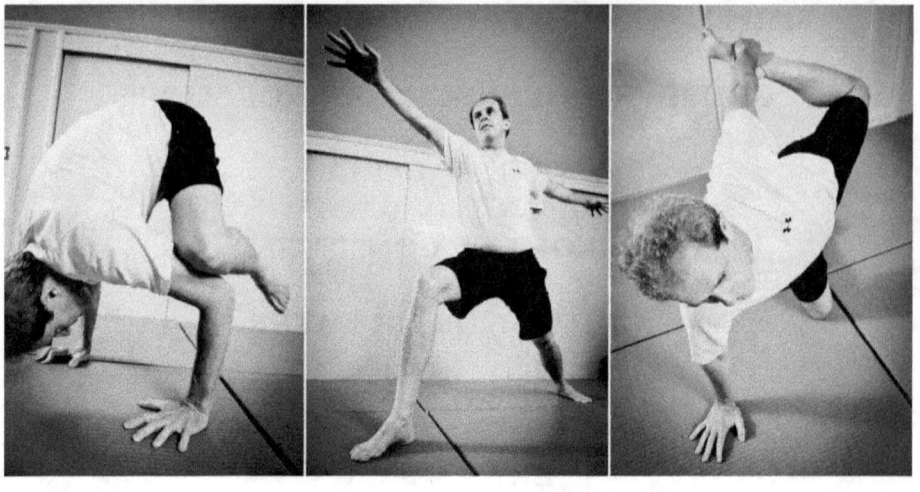

Workouts that emphasize flexibility are also important. Stretching should be an integral part of any workout. Frequent practice will increase your natural flexibility at a normal rest rate. **A cold stretch is a light stretch used to loosen your muscles.** Examples include a light stretch after getting out of bed or a quick stretch after long periods of inactivity. More intense, prolonged stretching should only be done after your muscles are warm and loose. It is beneficial to stretch at different times throughout the day to reduce soreness and stiffness. Flexible people are more comfortable overall, because they are less likely to get injured.

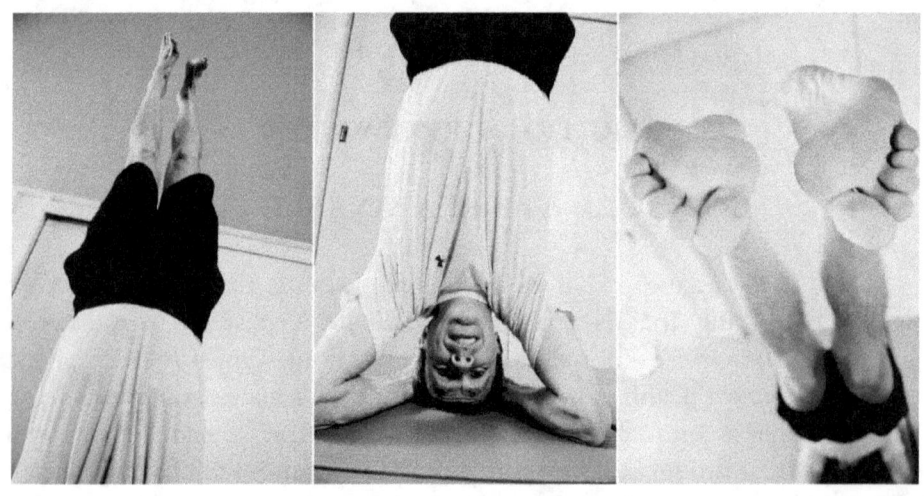

This means every morning wake up and do something, cold stretch, workout, or rest (if you're too sore from working out the day before). Ah, yes, resting is part of working out! When you rest you see greater gains, allow your muscles to recover and also get to appreciate the other wonderful things life has to offer. Eat right; we will go into this in further detail later. However, you get out of your body what you put into your body. If you are eating junk then that is what you are going to get out of your workouts, JUNK! If you are eating the right amount of vegetables, carbohydrates, protein, and fiber then.....well you get the idea.

Trained 2 B Tip

Potassium is essential for the proper functioning of the heart, kidneys, muscles, nerves, and digestive system, it is essential to get rid of lactic acid. Don't like bananas? (Neither do I) try potato's, spinach, sweet potatoes, yogurt, raisins, broccoli (love it) cantaloupe and peaches.

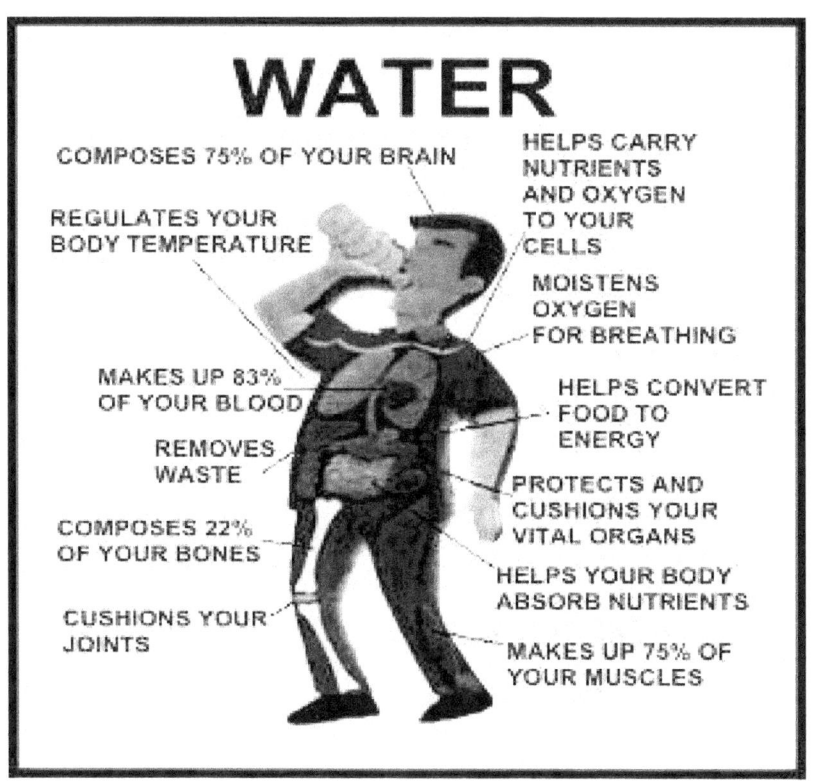

The Life Sensei's quick tips

Drinking water is also repeated on the list!

Drinking plenty of water will help to prevent bloating. It's difficult to realistically eliminate salt from your diet, but do try to limit the intake and balance it with plenty of water. Also, use sea salt as it is less refined and contains necessary trace minerals. The reason one retains water has to do with hormones. A high salt concentration will trigger it to make you retain water, and therefore you will be bloated. Water not only decreases appetite, it prevents those "hungry horror moments" we all encounter when our blood sugar drops and we reach for cookies, candy, ice cream, fries or other high-calorie treats. Water also cleans out the system, rids the body of toxins, helps keep your complexion looking healthy, and allows the body to function at its best. Nothing quells the appetite like water.

Start out with two bottles in the morning and carry one with you to work or wherever you go. If you like, divvy up the 64 ounces of water into eight (8-ounce) bottles or four pint (16-ounce) bottles to carry around with you all day. Freeze half of them the night before and they will last all day, even in a hot car. Keep some unfrozen so they will be ready to drink immediately. If you do not like the taste get over it, or try some flavored water. Some studies have indicated that you can actually drink too much water. Your body will tell you when it's had enough. Likewise you should not have pain or develop swelling from drinking water.

What runs but never gets tired? Water

Ok, corny jokes aside the answer should be you!

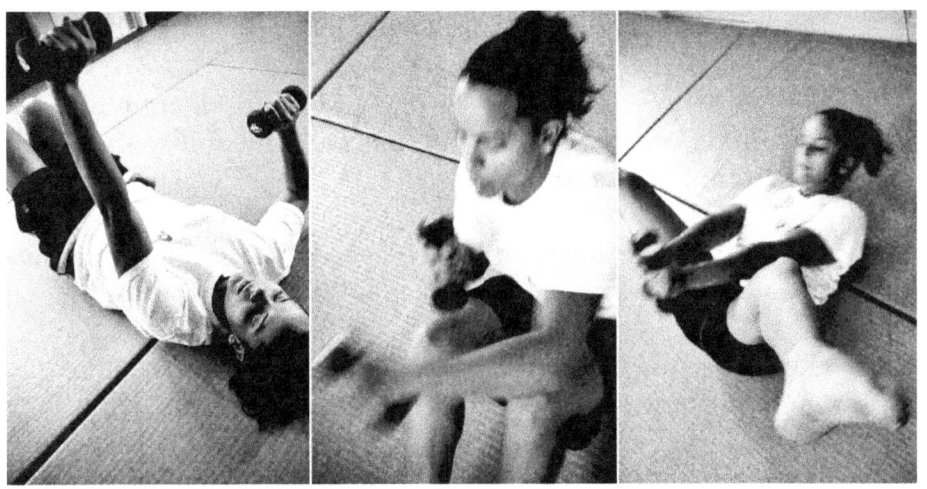

Building consistency

Being consistent is the meat and potatoes of realistic fitness goals. First off, everyone should work out every day. **Consistency is defined as firmness of constitution or character. Look at it as the more consistent you are, the stronger your backside, thighs, abs, and triceps will be.** The more consistent you are the more focused your character will be. Your ability to resist temptation, in all forms, will be stronger and more reliable. Your body will be less prone to injury. If you do get injured, you will heal faster. Your recovery time will be less. You will fit into your dress or jeans more often. You can run around with your children. They, in turn, will follow your lead.

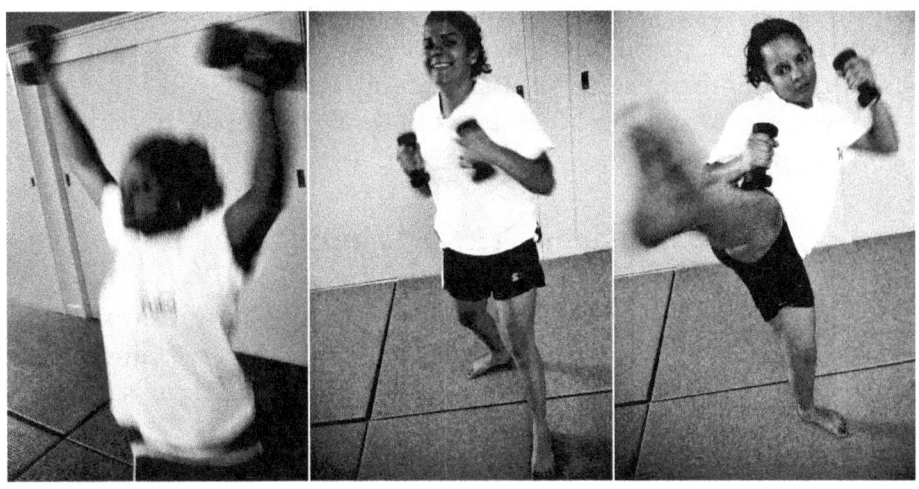

The Life Sensei's quick tips

Try to incorporate both cardio and strength training into your workouts. Core/ abdominal strength and flexibility should be implemented in both workouts.

Cardio can be anything that uses the large body muscles and keeps your heart rate elevated over short periods of time.

Running, bicycling, treadmills, step machines, kickboxing, swimming, power walking, are all great exercises.

Strength training is necessary to promote muscle growth, which increases endurance and stamina and overall calorie burn.

Weightlifting and resistance training are examples. Your core/abs training will assist in improving your overall conditioning.

The stability ball can be used for abdominal and lower back exercises, and Pilates based abs routines works well also.

TRUTH

Understand that getting in shape requires commitment and a realistic game plan. Grab a dedicated partner and incorporate cardio, strength training, and stretching into your routines. Make sure you put the right fuel in your body to keep the machine working properly.

The Life Sensei says, "Think about it"

According to the Consumer Products Safety Commission, 50,000 people a year visit emergency room due to injury while exercising. Get a trainer, avoid DVD's, and machine's without proper supervision.

The Life Sensei on Cardio

Pre workout Cardio and Cardio tips

The key to sticking with a cardiovascular routine is picking an activity that you really enjoy doing.

Start every training session with 5-15 minutes of cardio. By doing the cardio before you train you will be able to increase your core temperature and thus be less likely to get injured while training.

Do the cardio interval style, going easy for 1 minute and then hard for one minute.

Whatever your chosen cardio activity is, having the right equipment is a must.

Music is a powerful motivator and can make time fly by, which will make your workouts feel finished before they've begun.

If you dislike doing cardio and are consistent when it comes to weight training; mix in a few minutes of cardio between sets.

Getting your cardio on when your body has used up much of its readily available energy is crucial. Your body is forced to use its energy reserves in order to get you through the cardio exercise.

Total body workouts are a must! With all the new trends don't forget that you want to be consistent and spend your time wisely.

If you don't push yourself, no one else will. No excuses, fight through your comfort zone and get it done.

Your body is what you put in to it, if you want to see better results you have to do cardiovascular exercises.

the LifeSensei Workout Challenge
bicep curls
tricep kickback
bent over row
shoulder press
lunges
squats
calf raises
farmers walk

:30 jumping jacks
:30 mountain climbers
:30 jump front kicks
in between each weight drill
theLifeSenSei.trainerze.com for the videos to exercises

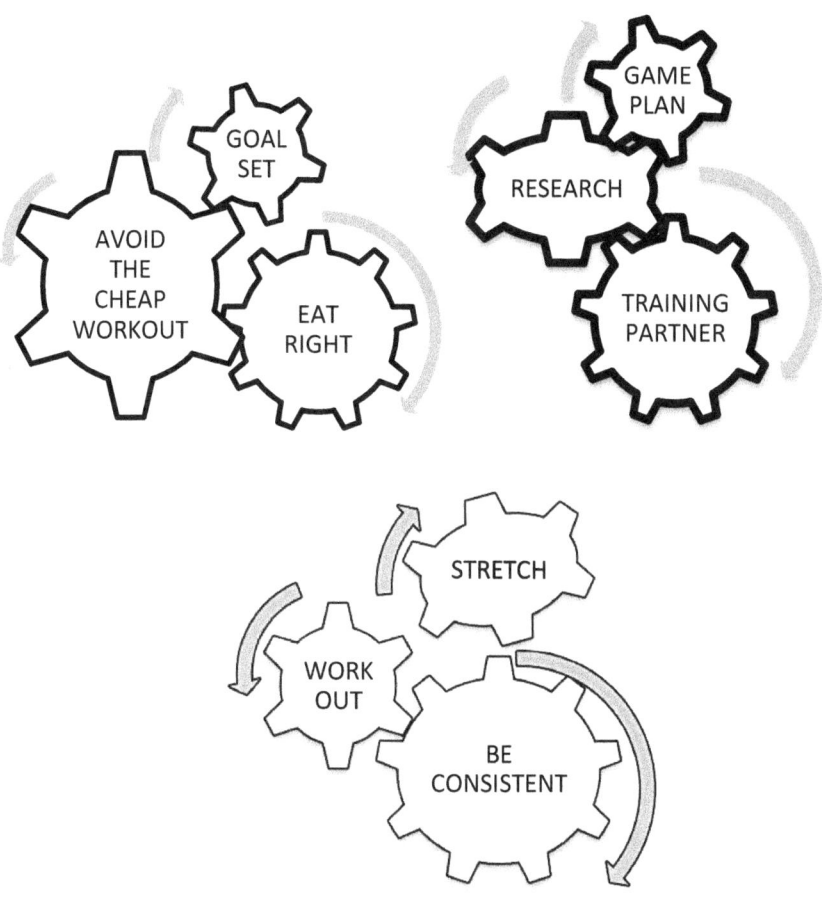

You are on your way to a new successful you!

The Life Sensei says, "Think about it"

How would you describe yourself? Where do you "fit"?

SIMPLE: Disregard all advice and go back to watching TV.

AVERAGE: Make an excuse, ANY EXCUSE.

GREAT! Goal Set, Game Plan, Find a partner (yeah right now).

BALANCE: Plan time to have fun, with your friends, family and enjoy your own company once in awhile.

The Life Sensei says, "Think about it"

If you do not get in the game, you won't really be playing. If you do not develop a game plan you cannot truly win.

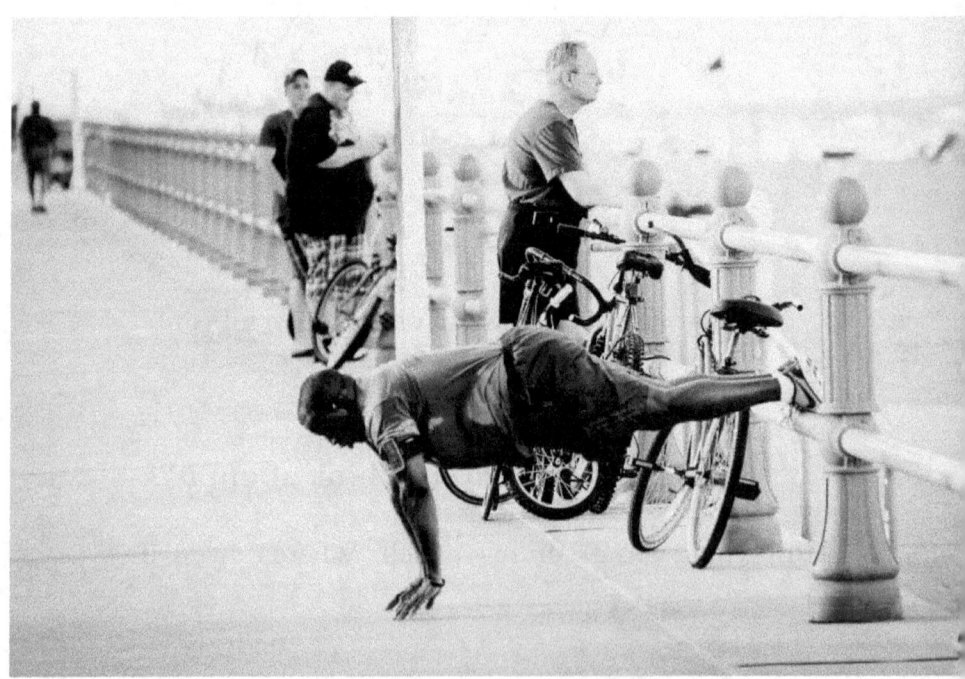

Martial guidance for life's journey

MYOFASCIAL STRETCHING	DYNAMIC STRETCHING	STATIC STRETCHING
USE A FOAM ROLLER TO APPLY PRESSURE TO DIFFERENT MUSCLES	WITHOUT HOLDING A POSITION MOVE LIMBS TO INCREASE RANGE	MUSCLES PAIN FREE FOR AS FAR AS YOU CAN FOR AS LONG AS YOU CAN
DO THIS ANYTIME YOU HAVE TIME!	BEFORE YOU WORK OUT BEFORE A CARDIO WARMUP	AFTER YOU WORKOUT DO NOT FORGET
GET RID OF KNOTS LESS TENSION	PREPARES BODY FOR WORKOUT BUILDS MUSCLE MEMORY	INCREASE YOUR FLEXIBILITY
PUT ALL YOUR BODY WEIGHT INTO IT IT PAYS OFF SO DO IT	REMAIN SMOOTH COOL AND CONTROLLED	HOLD FOR 30 SECONDS IMPROVE TIME AS YOU GET BETTER

One song workout part 1

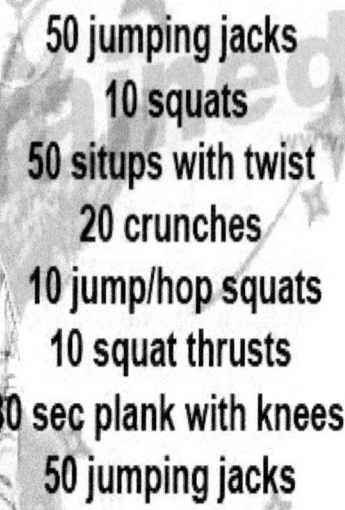

50 jumping jacks
10 squats
50 situps with twist
20 crunches
10 jump/hop squats
10 squat thrusts
:30 sec plank with knees
50 jumping jacks

theLifeSenSei.trainerze.com for the videos to exercises

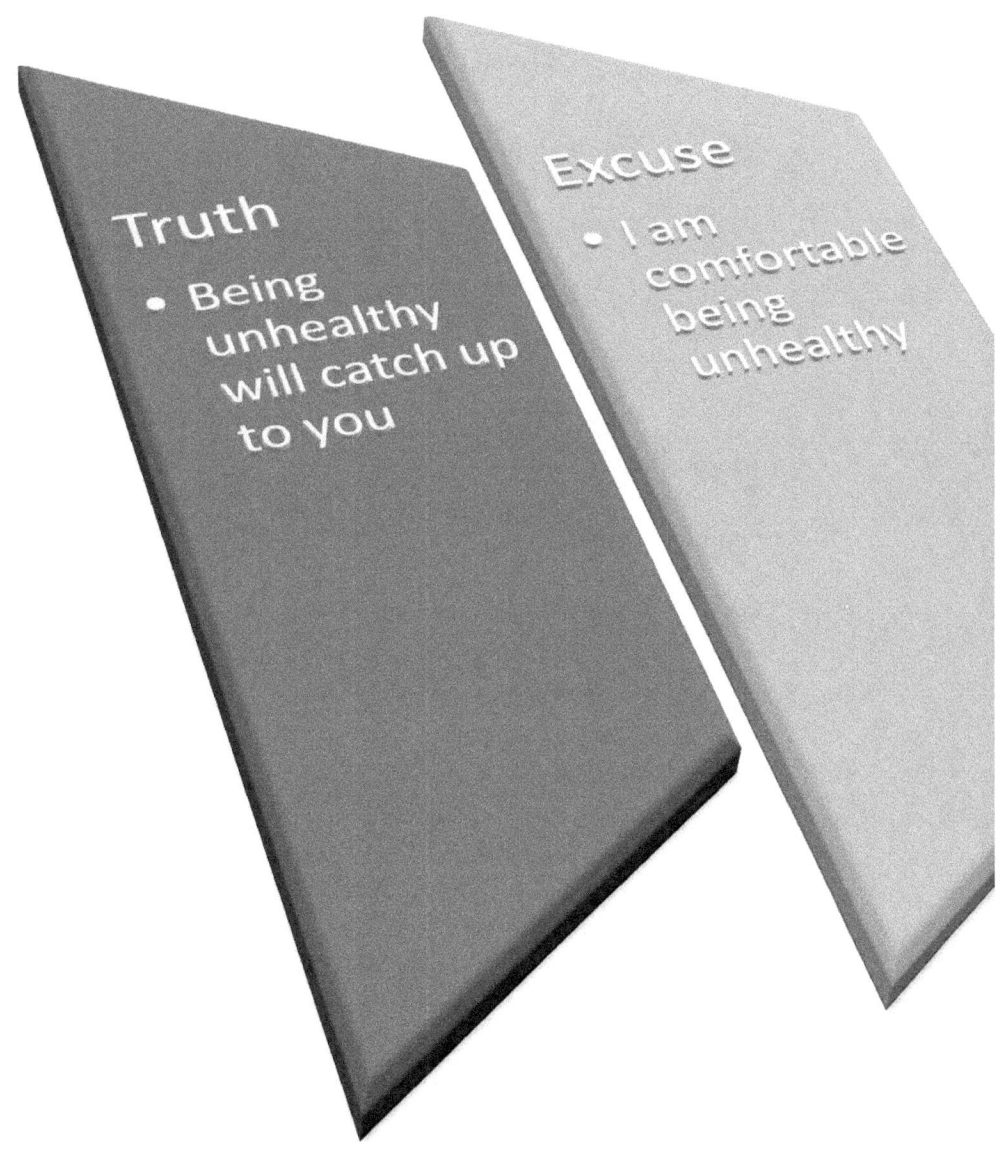

Truth
- Being unhealthy will catch up to you

Excuse
- I am comfortable being unhealthy

Plan

Instead of Soda, Coffee and Alcohol try water

Instead of Pizza, Fried Foods and Junk Foods try salads

You can add supplements to the water or proteins to the salad

Implement

Time, Money, Power, Respect

We cannot control any of these things

So manage yours responsibly

Habit

Road Rage, Flipping the Bird, Losing Control

When you do it you are only teaching others to do the same

Slow down, give the thumbs up, or calm yourself

Result

Stairs

Before the elevator was created

A flight of stairs helped to keep one fit

Take every opportunity to use them

To keep your legs and cardio in shape

When that gets easy, run up the steps

3rd Stop: *Get in Shape & Stay in Shape*

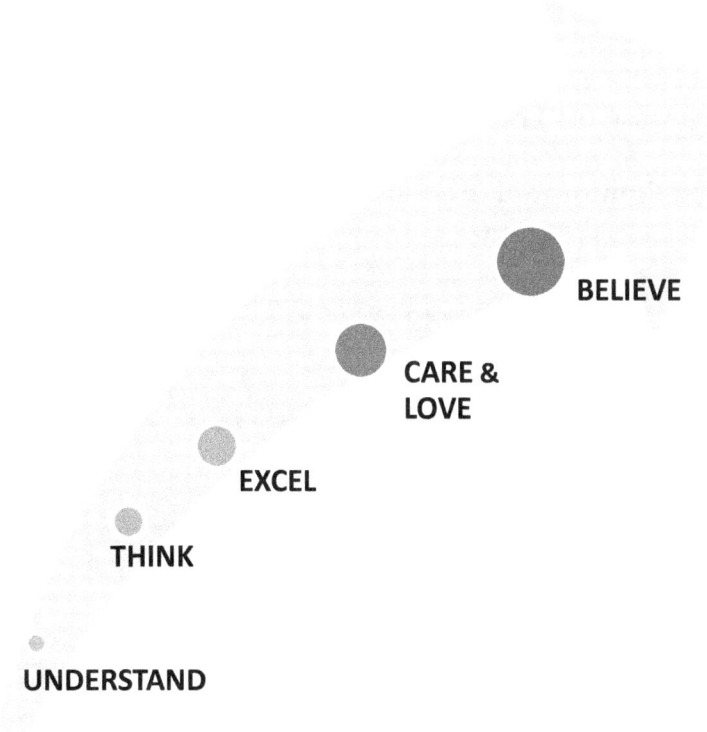

Are you trained to be the <u>BEST</u> you possible?

"Live life with love, caring for others, and understand what makes us different. Believe in yourself, conquer problems and overcome setbacks. Excel to be the best you possible." -Sensei Mitchell

"2 Believe"- Put your faith in to action

"Only you can do it, but you can't do it alone." unknown author

Whatever you believe, do it earnestly with conscious thoughts and a cheerful heart. Regardless of what you believe, you have a choice. You can choose to put what you believe into action or you can choose to ignore what you believe. If you believe something, but do not stay true to your beliefs, then you are in conflict with yourself. Your spirit knows what you believe, even if mentally you do not acknowledge it. When people do what they know is right, they won't be in conflict.

Straightforward example: Not knowing what to believe in, feeling empty and confused.

Universal example: Following your parents or peers beliefs, at face value

Complicated example: Finding what you believe in through life lessons, putting your faith into action.

Training 2 believe is standing up not just for what you may believe is right or wrong, just or unjust, but to actually stand up!

Training to believe in yourself can help you keep your diet, wake up in the morning and stretch. In turn you will eat better, focus longer, train harder. It can allow you to make the right decisions involving your health, lifestyle and belief system. Faith in others allows you to see the good in people, which can strengthen the trust and dependency in relationships. Share your beliefs with likeminded people, who in turn will put their faith in you. Putting your faith into action helps you plan successfully. This makes it easier to fulfill your goals, inspiring you to create new challenges. When you set the events in motion, knowing that someone is in your corner is the best feeling in the world. However, you still need to believe in yourself, since no one else can believe in you better than ….you.

"There may be times where you cannot find help, but never a time where you cannot give it." -unknown author

Learning to care for others helps you take better care of yourself. By recognizing that there is always someone more in need, you can better appreciate what you have. Some people would give anything to live in your shoes. Surely they would take care of their bodies to ensure they can do all the things they've always wanted to do but perhaps could not. You are looking for ways to motivate yourself, to get off of your backside and get in shape. You're looking for reasons to take care of yourself and they are right in front of you. Motivate yourself! Get your life straight, put your affairs in order, and live the life you want to live.

Trained 2 care: by helping others you end up helping yourself. Start a Runner or Walker's club with your neighbors. Get the community together and paint a mural (which burns calories while building relationships). Invite a friend who is going through rough times to hit a heavy bag with you at the gym. Offer to assist someone with the groceries weekly, and use the shopping bags as weights. Start a charity event that requires push-ups, sit-ups or another physical activity for a worthy cause. The desire to care and create change is inside of you. Let it out today!

The Life Sensei says, "Think about it"

If you want to get anything out of life, you have to give. My grandmother says, "You cannot get anything if your hand is closed".

"2 Excel" - U were created uniquely, B the best U every day

"Inside of you lie dreams unrealized, goals not completed, countries never visited and relationships lost, instruments waiting to be played. What are you waiting for?" -Sensei Mitchell

You excel because you plan, implement and execute your dreams.

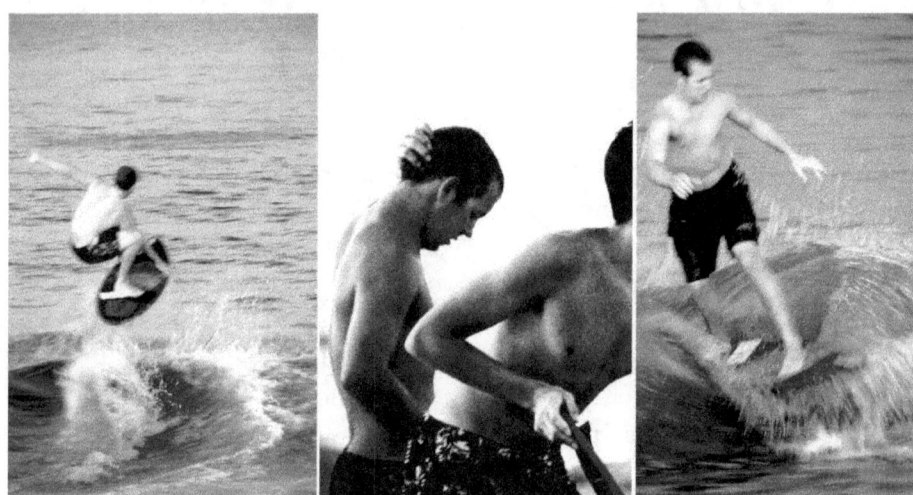

Train 2 excel: by not only setting a goal but raising the bar so that when you reach your goal you are outstanding!

- You go to school not just to get a better job, but to enjoy your life to the fullest.
- You are looking for that special someone not to get married and have kids, but to have the best possible family and life-mate ever.
- You play sports because you love the game, are consumed by it and want to play at the highest level competing for the highest championship.
- You want to get and stay in shape. Once you reach your goal you are going to set new ones, like doing something fun with that new body of yours: traveling, modeling, competing, and going out more.

When you train to excel, you eat right, study longer, rest and set realistic goals. Track your progress; find likeminded people to accelerate your growth. You listen to solid advice even when you do not want to. You are constantly pushing your limits and discovering there is more to you than even you realized. You do not just play sports, you dominate them. You take tests and make them look easy. You work hard and play hard. You motivate, and inspire others regardless of job, age, or what others may foolishly look at as setbacks. You see that your dreams are your way of telling you what will make you happy. You listen to them and make them real.

Do what makes you happy... the best are not the happiest but the happiest are usually the best.

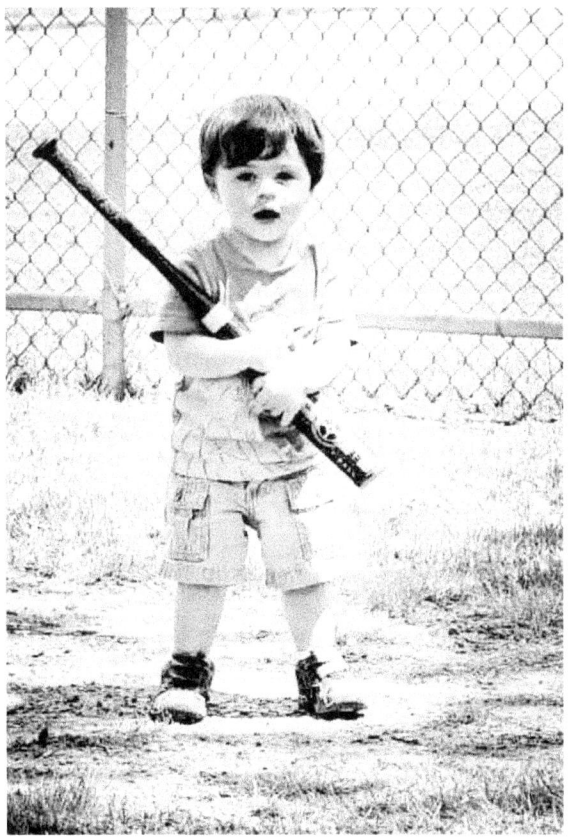

Never let go of your dreams and set your ambitions high!

"2 Love" - Test your love by your love for one another

"If you love, you respect others and yourself. If you do not love, you do not respect anything..."-Sensei Mitchell

Love is the commandment for fulfilling all commandments & the rule for fulfilling all rules.

If you don't do these things, you owe it to yourself, your family and friends to find out why.

Trained 2 love is eating the right foods, working out that extra day, treating yourself to a personal training session, getting a massage, (getting your nails done doesn't count, unless it's a treat not a regular visit). Buy yourself something nice, take yourself out, buy a book, or go to the movies. Buy yourself a ticket to one of your favorite shows. Trained to love is accepting and learning to understand things that are different from you. It is giving your loved ones verbal affirmation and showing it through actions daily. Trained to love is losing extra weight the right way or accepting your body for what it is, yours. Trained 2 love is standing up for yourself, speaking your mind, seeing yourself succeed before you even begin something. Trained 2 love is being able to love yourself, no one can do that as well as you!

Loving merely requires that you put others before yourself.

Take a conscious effort to reflect on your actions before you act.

Learn to create positive habits where your love is seen.

When in doubt, love more.

"2 Think" - Instruction ends with school, education ends with life

"Do not be misinformed; pursue knowledge, seek truth, and find proof"- Sensei Mitchell

Trained 2 Think:

- Are you still improving your knowledge base?
- Is personal experience your only teacher, or do you seek other forms of enlightenment?
- Do you believe everything you hear and read, do you check to see if what you are told is true?
- Do you question, or do you let your suspicions go unanswered?
- Are you free to speak your mind, or are you afraid others won't understand and ostracize you?
- Are you a spark for others or are you detrimental to others thinking?
- Do you allow others to grow, are you mentoring someone?

Trained 2 think, is taking the time to educate yourself and others. It's reviewing information and using it to make solid decisions. Trained to think is writing, journaling, reading, improving and updating what you already know. It's taking the time to consistently, and positively educate our children. It's taking the time to answer questions about sex, gangs, drugs and life; honestly sharing your knowledge. It's sharing your experiences or honestly reviewing history. Trained 2 think does not mean believing everything you hear.

Trained 2 think is watching what you eat and setting realistic goals. It is thinking before you speak and actively listening before you react. It's taking your trainer's advice and applying it. It's putting that dessert back in the fridge or better yet, throwing it away. It's making a plan in advance so that you can be ahead of the game. Trained to think is being aware of where your children are *and* what they are doing. Better than that, it's enrolling them in a program or participating with them in activities. It's staying away from the scale, because you know what you weigh; since you're following your diet.

"If ignorance is bliss why aren't more people jumping up for joy?"
unknown author

Life is challenging enough. Do not let fear, ignorance, and hatred or jealously set you further back. Educate yourself so you can relate to yourself. Then you can relate to others regardless of the color of skin, lifestyle, preferences, mistakes, or differences.

Straightforward example: You are ignorant, your lack of understanding results in unrealistic expectations, fears and actions. Worse than being unaware you're comfortable with your ignorance.

Universal example: Following your parents or peers beliefs, at face value has made you racist, prideful and anti-social with people who are different than you. It's easier to just conform than make a change.

Complicated example: Finding out what you believe in through life lessons, personal experiences and challenging yourself enough to look past obvious differences others find easy to point out.

This Chapter was designed to educate, develop open and honest dialogue for those uncomfortable or unable to speak for themselves: We need fit minds as well as bodies!

The Life Sensei says, "Think about it"

"Be conscious of your choices & be responsible for your action."

"The greatest gift you can give you somebody is your own personal development. I used to say, "If you will take care of me, I will take care of you."Now I say, I will take care of me for you, if you will take care of you for me." Jim Rohn

Being Trained 2 understand is not easy, nor should it be; our Earth is now home to over 6.7 billion people. This year, 73 million people will be added to the planet, and by the year 2050, the United Nations projects that the world's population will be between 7.8 and 10.5 billion (give or take). So honestly, it is difficult to relate to everyone because we are all individuals; unique and different. But we should respect and love each other since we are all human.

- We all breathe the same air, drink the same water, and live on the same planet.
- We all have ancestry on this planet and can be linked to one original family.
- We all live and die the same, what is different is how we choose to live.
- We all have had struggles, hardships and have triumphantly continued on.
- We all are worthy of a second chance, entitled to making a mistake, deserving of being forgiven.
- We all have a past we would rather forget, a moment we wish we can take back.
- We all might sometimes wish we can turn back the clock of time and live life over.
- We all want to be loved, respected and desire something better for our loved ones and our self.

Training 2 understand, is seeing you in others, learning to not pass judgment. Its educating yourself to understand what makes us unique and different. It's doing your best to be an ambassador of the human race, the only race that really matters.

TRUTH

Trained 2 B is not a choice; it's a way of life. To some degree everybody needs to improve. If you put others before yourself, make sure it's for the right reasons. If you put yourself before others, make sure it's to make yourself healthier. If you do not do these things you will be searching for a peace that you may never find, alienating and hurting the people you should care about.

Waist Trimmer

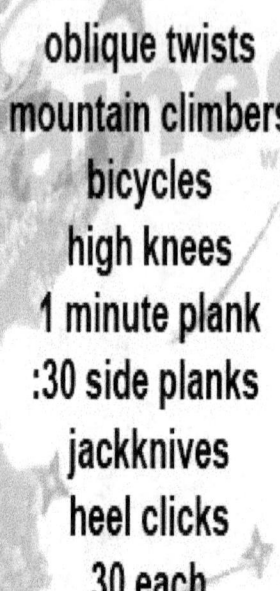

oblique twists

mountain climbers

bicycles

high knees

1 minute plank

:30 side planks

jackknives

heel clicks

30 each

repeat for 3 minutes

work up to 5 minutes daily

theLifeSenSei.trainerze.com for the videos to exercises

The Life Sensei says "Think about it"

There is no substitute for doing the right thing. Besides legal issues, only you can determine what is right or wrong for yourself. But, everyone inside knows the difference between right or wrong. So if you complain that your life is out of order, or you are waiting for things to set themselves straight take a look at the "man in the mirror" first and "don't be cruel."

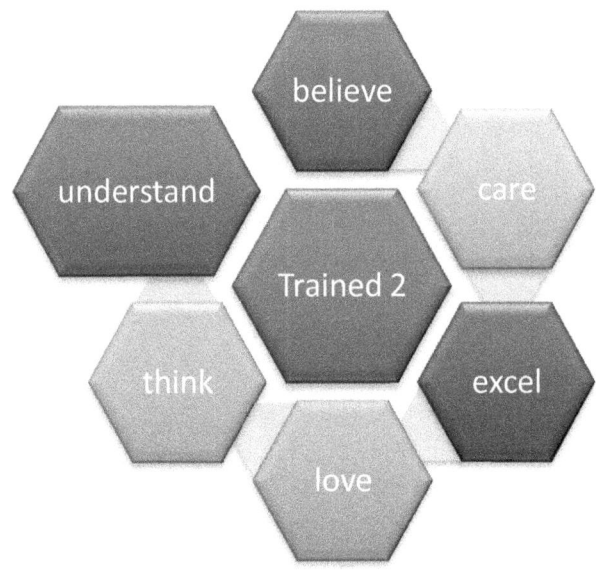

SIMPLE: Continue living with fear, hate, quitters' attitude, ignorance and unbelief, see how much further that gets you.

AVERAGE: Attend services because you have to follow everything someone tells you to do because it's easier. Trust the powers that be; they always have your best interest at heart. Do not be concerned with the details. You only have one life to live.

GREAT! : Read the chapter and apply it. I promise it will spark a change in you, which will light the path to a better you.

BALANCE: Put yourself in the life you are quick to judge, how would you like to be treated?

The Life Sensei on "Why we get fat?"

It all begins with perspective.

When we are comfortable with our place in life; our weight, health, money and time do not have numbers behind it.

We look at our relationships, paychecks, status and because we feel like we are in a good place we don't feel the need to evolve.

We find ourselves happy initially, with our family, friends, loved ones, coworkers but as we continue to grow old we realize something is missing.

We let ourselves go, it doesn't matter what size you are, how much weight you put on or you have lost.

"Fat" doesn't have to mean excess skin, it could be bad habits in any shape or form that get in the way of your health.

Don't get to comfortable in a relationship, especially in regards to the one you have with your body. Your body will trade perceived happiness for a decline in health starting with an accumulation of "fat".

It ends with reality.

As we become uncomfortable with our place in life; at any moment our weight, health, money and time begin to have numbers attached.

We are now watching these numbers and can't seem to find the resolve or the interest in making those numbers disappear again.

So we ignore them, and hope without working, try without committing and fail to see how our perspective becomes our reality.

That's why we get fat.

Martial guidance for life's journey

Stop Stress!

Relax every day. Deep-belly breathing, meditation and sleeping are all tried-and-true ways to beat stress.

The best workout is one that includes the mind and spirit as well as the body. Consider some alternatives to your weight and cardio training. Include these mind/body disciplines on a regular basis and feel the difference.

Give volunteer work a try. It's a great way to take your mind off your own troubles and it gives you a great sense of accomplishment when you volunteer your time and energy to a good cause.

Go outside and move. You've heard it before, but daily exercise is one of the best stress reducers you'll ever find and it will also help you lose weight. Also, pick one thing you have been putting off such as scheduling an appointment, running an errand, or returning a phone call, saying you're sorry and do it immediately. Taking care of one nagging responsibility can be revitalizing and can improve your overall attitude.

For every one hour of work, take a five minute break and stretch, walk, or meditate. With just a few minutes of relaxation (or doing something other than work), you'll increase your physical activity as well as productivity and feel better throughout the day creating a positive habit. Limit stress-fueled pigging out. People who frequently turn to food when stressed have higher levels of both insulin and can get diabetes later on in life.

Think positively. Negative thought patterns create stress, but if you learn to look on the bright side more, you can cut tension. Go back through this book which is filled with tips on how to improve your outlook and fight negative thinking.

Stress Less

dance it out

go for a walk (bring a dog)

talk about it

breathe

go to bed earlier

focus on what you can do

ask for a hug

give a hug

look for moments to be great

smile

smile more

theLifeSenSei.trainerze.com for the videos to exercises

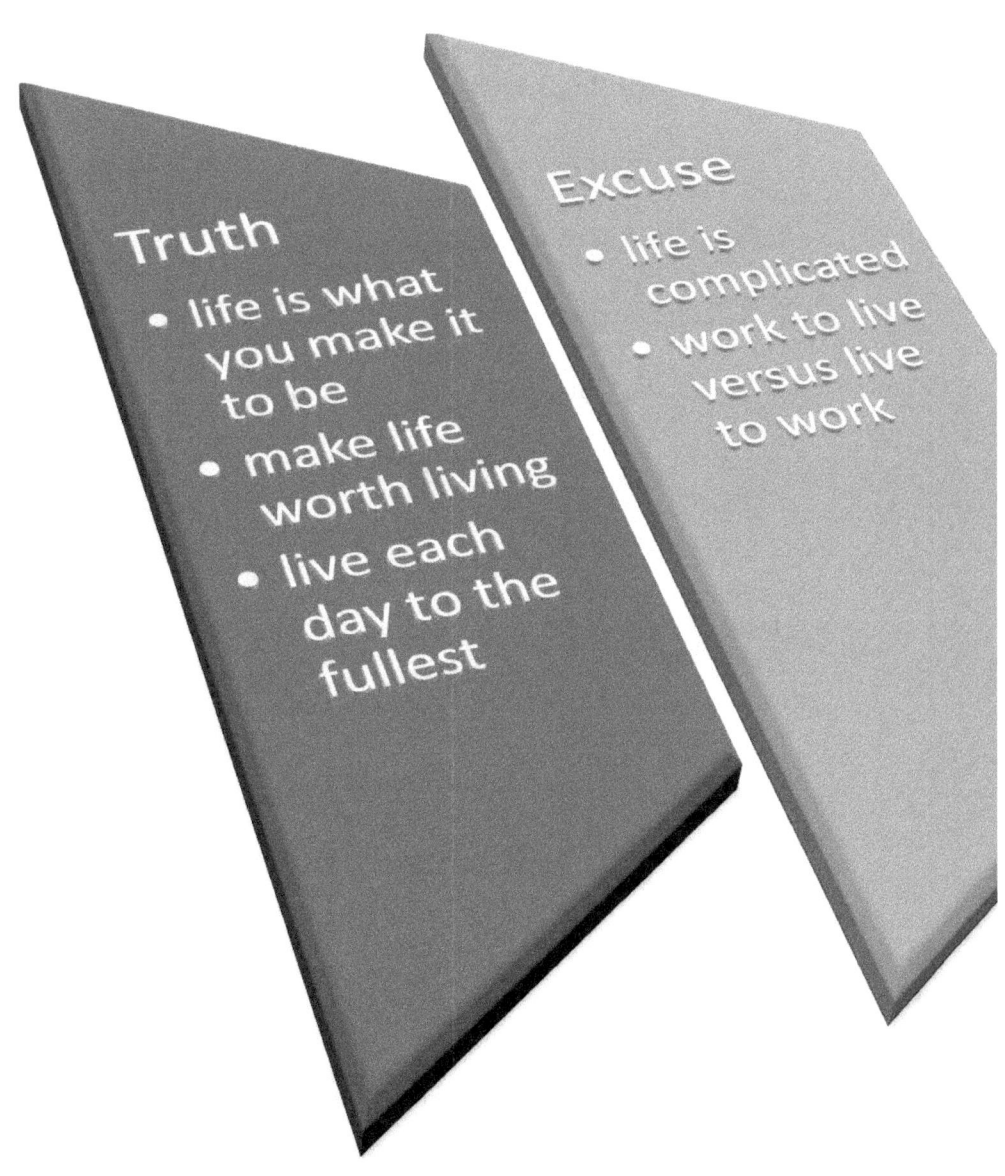

Truth
- life is what you make it to be
- make life worth living
- live each day to the fullest

Excuse
- life is complicated
- work to live versus live to work

Plan

Do Lose: weight, excuses, fat

Do Not Lose: time, money, muscle

Implement

TRAINED: to form by instruction, discipline, or drill

To make prepared (as by exercise) for a test of skill

To teach so as to make fit, qualified, or proficient

To undergo instruction, discipline, or drill

To aim at an object or objective

Habit

Focus on your Happiness

Health, Job, Relationships, Age, Social Skills, Finances

Be at peace with your decisions

Focus on the Positive

Results

Dumbbells

Total Body Workout, Boxing, Kickboxing, Weight Lifting

Incorporate into your daily routine to build muscle definition

4th Stop: *Event for the Entire Family*

Working out is no longer an option

If all things are created equal, then is it better to be in shape than not in shape. That seems like common sense right? Yet, now obesity, gaining weight, and losing weight incorrectly are the norm for many people. All things unfortunately, are not created equal. At the end of the day, you have to be comfortable in your own skin. You have to be able to look past the hard moments during each day and look forward to the future. Until someone builds a time machine, you are not going to be able to do anything about yesterday.

If the past bothers you, do something about it today so that your tomorrow will be better.

Learn from each experience: grow, prepare, think, understand, and excel. You cannot change how people feel about you or what someone might think about you. Especially, if they are not willing to open themselves up to you. You **can** change how you feel and what you think about yourself. As much as I believe your change starts from within, some people still determine their self-worth by their appearance. Think about the bathing suit when it was first created. It used to cover your entire body. Today there are many different styles of bathing suits to choose. What changed from the first bathing suit to Speedos and thongs (or the birthday suit)? If modesty, nudity, protection from the elements was such an issue, when did it become socially acceptable to wear next to nothing? We fret about what we are going to wear to the beach or pool when the weather gets warm. We wear t-shirts or shorts to cover our chests, arms, stomachs, thighs and backside hiding what we feel is less than desirable.

"The older you get, the tougher it is to lose weight because by then, your body and your fat are really good friends." -Anonymous

Why are there gyms all over the place and I can't seem to get in shape?

Today it seems a new gym opens every year (at least); it has the best equipment, the juice bar, stunning personal trainers and all the quick fix clients it can handle. In all of your excitement, you miss out on the fine print where all the fixings cost more, like the juice bar, personal trainer, or weight loss advice. The gym is so cute and cuddly, you sign up with your girlfriend, sibling, best friend, coworker, mom, dad and dog. It is right around the corner from where you live so you can either crawl back in bed to skip a workout, or crawl out of bed if you decide to train. They offer low rates to draw you in, knowing that you will not stay committed and will not mind paying the low rate after you quit. Your contract with the gym has begun, so you jump head first believing that in 4 weeks to 3 months your old body will be transformed into the new you.

Your initial passion has you eating better or at least thinking about eating better. You begin to watch shows, read books, and listen more attentively to advice on getting in better shape. Friends now know better than to tempt you with dessert or fattening food. Your optimistic attitude is contagious. Your coworkers and family are wondering what has gotten into you. As you sleep better, the soreness in your muscles becomes unnoticeable. You stare in the mirror at the new body in front of you. Wondering why you have not begun working out sooner, you begin to take more classes enjoying how others are now looking at you differently. You feel capable, are thinking positively and hear the birds sing outside until….

A) **You weigh yourself**
B) **The jeans or business suit still doesn't fit right**
C) **Someone calls you fat or notices your belly**
D) **You miss a day, week or month and have to start all over**

"While we are making up our minds as to when we shall begin the opportunity is lost." -unknown author

Seem familiar? Do you sense that wacky, annoying feeling that you are never going to reach your goals? Do you feel as if no one is going to notice that change in your body? Are you concerned your outfits will not fit, and you cannot get back to the proper shape you had when you were younger? You used to be able to lift so much more weight, run faster, and bend lower. What happened? Maybe you were never that flexible, hated sports and never saw the benefits of working out. Maybe you were a model or were always in shape without doing anything; now you notice the effect of everything you eat, on your body.

Maybe you had an injury and hesitated to get back in shape. You might have even played on a team earlier in your life and it drives you insane you are not the same athlete. If you never worked out before, you may be wondering why in the world you should start now. It feels as if you are going after unattainable goals for the rest of your life.

As the days go by, you wonder why your personal trainer does not pay as much attention to you anymore. That cardio instructor does not help you stretch. You realize for the amount of money you spend on the juice bar you can buy a juice machine making your own drinks. Your frustration grows as your friend's stop going with you to workout. On top of that, you still aren't seeing the results you want and you are the third person in line for the elliptical machine.

Now those diet pills are beginning to look more enticing to you, since that wedding is coming up and you do not want your peers to look better than you. You pay more attention to those diet fads and quick weight loss meals because something has to give. You wonder if plastic surgery would work for you, or if steroids are that pathetic after all. You get annoyed when your instructor is pushing you harder. You know that he has your best interest in mind, but it does not matter to you. That guy/girl that started training after you looks terrific and seems to be losing weight faster. The people that used to stop and stare seem to look the other way when you enter the room.

Wondering what you were thinking in the first place, you sleep in rather than attend your private training sessions. You skip stretching during your favorite TV show and sabotage eating habits by binging. You secretly start building a voodoo doll to torment anyone that gets in your way. You are angry not only because you have not fulfilled your dream by reaching your goal, but because you feel as if it was never attainable. Your problems all started when you joined that gym for only a few bucks a month so you quit.

Besides, who wants to acknowledge that they are not seeing results? Eventually, you lose faith in the gym, rationalizing that it was not for you in the first place. These new gyms represent the future of working out in America; pay us for results. If you have money, we will do everything in our power to help you look and feel fabulous; if you do not well you are on your own. How many times do you have to rejoin a gym until you realize your current method of losing and maintaining weight is not working?

This new trend works because you have become so accustomed to paying nothing for nothing. You pay next to nothing to train at the gym and so you receive… next to nothing. Sure, you felt passionate after you lost your initial weight (congratulations) but, now it has been six months and you have plateau or have gone backwards. Everybody likes to get something for nothing: Free music, gifts, advice. Nobody likes to give away stuff for free. What people don't realize is that the businesses have caught on. Low price, low product is the new deal.

Where have you learned this behavior and why is it affecting your workouts?

- when you learned to settle instead of wanting the best
- when you allow others to determine what you are worth
- when you accepted failure as an option
- when you decided that your needs and happiness weren't that important

The Life Sensei's quick tips

As your priorities become clearer to you, the choices that you make become less about what you want and more about what you need. As you begin to realize that what you want is not what you need, you subconsciously begin to expect and demand more of yourself and less of others.

1. Who wants to admit that working out is hard, full of trials and errors?

2. Who wants to admit that they are not doing all they can to reach their goals?

3. Who wants to admit that they have settled, are not comfortable or have gone as far as they could?

Now you will not spend more money on yourself for a personal trainer, a weight loss plan, or to train at a more expensive gym since you cannot put a value on what you were paying for at the lower priced gym. You may say it's easy for a gym owner to say that, but believe it is not. My comments on the subject will leave me isolated or ostracized from most of my peers. They do not pay my bills or have to sleep in my bed. They do not have to look at my face in the mirror so I'm alright with that. Jerry Maguire was a movie about doing the right thing even if it was not the conventional thing. As long as I do not have to walk out of an office with just my fish and secretary, I'm happy. Bottom line, the truth is the truth.

What you are looking for is a gym where you are not just a number, where your questions get answered and where everyone who trains regularly sees results. You are looking for a gym where your money and time is valued, where instead of new products and equipment you get reliable instruction and consistent results instead. You are looking for a gym where everyone is treated equally, where the workouts are challenging and creative. Where the advice given is knowledgeable and real, positive attitudes are infectious and inspiring. A place where you are missed if you have not shown in a week or a month and when you receive a phone call it is not for more money.

Think about the outdoor walkers, joggers and runners who get up every morning regardless of the weather to workout. What is their motivation? Who gets up before them to wake them up? Who reminds them that they are doing a superb job and how much money are they spending for their results? Who motivates those who rollerblade, bicycle and jump rope? Who motivates those who attack the pavement outside with the wind blowing in their face? How about those who wake up and stretch, doing pushups, sit-ups, squats and so forth, from the comfort of their home without a gym membership?

Everyone is different. There are some who need gyms and others who do not. There are people who need motivation and others who hate having someone yelling in their face. For every person, who loves a class with instruction there are others who love to see the open road or lake instead of a gym atmosphere. The common denominator is, these people are doing something for themselves to ensure they are in the best shape possible. What are you doing? Are you limited due to lack of time, motivation and money?

The Life Sensei says, "Think about it"

You get what you pay for

Here is a little known fact about those who are wealthy and those who are not. The rich do not purchase cheap products. You will not find them driving a lower-priced, out-of-style vehicle or carrying a counterfeit bag. If you have to ask how much something costs, then to the wealthy it is too expensive for you. They do not shop at malls they shop at boutiques. They do not follow trends, they start them. Most importantly, they do not care what they look like because they are filthy rich. They go from being skinny to fat and blonde to brunette in a year. They have breast implants, breast reductions and wear trendy sunglasses depending on their mood simply because they can. They can afford the luxuries the average person cannot (Please understand I am generalizing to make a point. Work with me, ok.)

Remember, usually the celebrity has more free time than the average person. They can cheat if they want or take days off if they want because they have more time to train than you. They can eat what they want and plan their workout according to their needs since someone is waiting on them and servicing them. They can also go see a surgeon and get the look that they want in a day or two for the right price and the general public will not be any wiser. Do you think the wealthy respond to $50 or less gym memberships that require you to sign up for a year? Maybe you think that those gyms target that income group also, like they targeted you. You are aware that you were sought to train at that gym because of your income, right?

When someone who has an abundance of extra spending money decides to work out, they often do it in the confines of their home. A trainer visits them and tells them what to do. They create new and fun variations of the same exercises. They push them gently and with purpose because otherwise the client will find another trainer. They take the time to convince the client that the drills are in their best interest and name drop other clients they have that have seen results. They cook for them using the finest foods and ingredients, preparing meals for them each day. They write journals or diaries to track their progress through conversations. They do not train in large classes where the attention of the trainer is everywhere and they pay for the session whether they are late, actually workout or just want to talk.

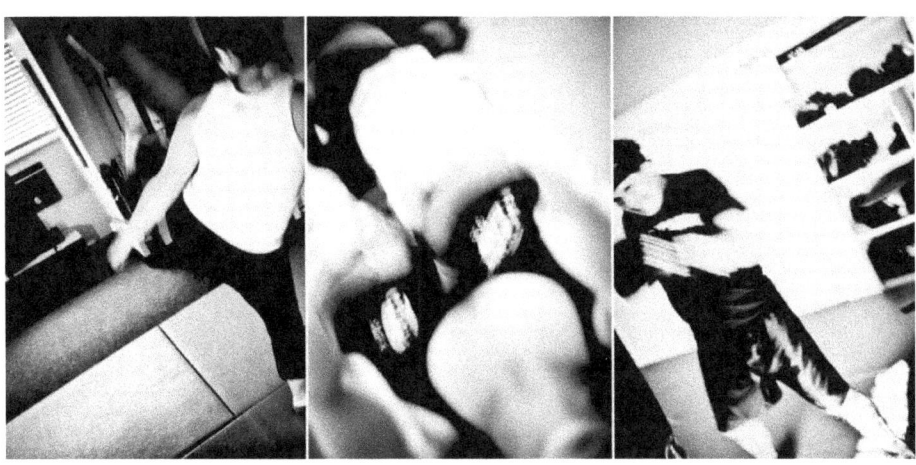

The Life Sensei's quick tips

1. If you had the money to train with a trainer, the best equipment to work with, and the time needed to get in the best shape ever would you?

2. What would you do differently from what you're doing now?

3. How would you feel if you saw results immediately?

4. Would you continue or stop?

5. Would you eat healthy or eat more junk food?

6. What would you do with your new body, would you flaunt it?

7. Are you better off at a gym working out at home or outside; maybe all three?

Think about it. Personal Trainers, Instructors and Coaches help you see results faster. For the right price you will either get in great shape or feel great about trying to get in great shape. (Conversely you can work with a trainer that can also make you feel and look worse for the right price; so do your homework).What are you paying for at your gym?

- Are you paying for the upkeep of the gym?
- Is your gym really attractive with all the fixings and amenities while you look the same?
- Is the newer equipment helping you reach goals or helping attract new members?
- Are you doing the same routine every day, week, and month and seeing the same results?
- Does your instructor or gym owner have your best interests in mind?
- Are you worth investing in and do you have to be rich to think like the rich?

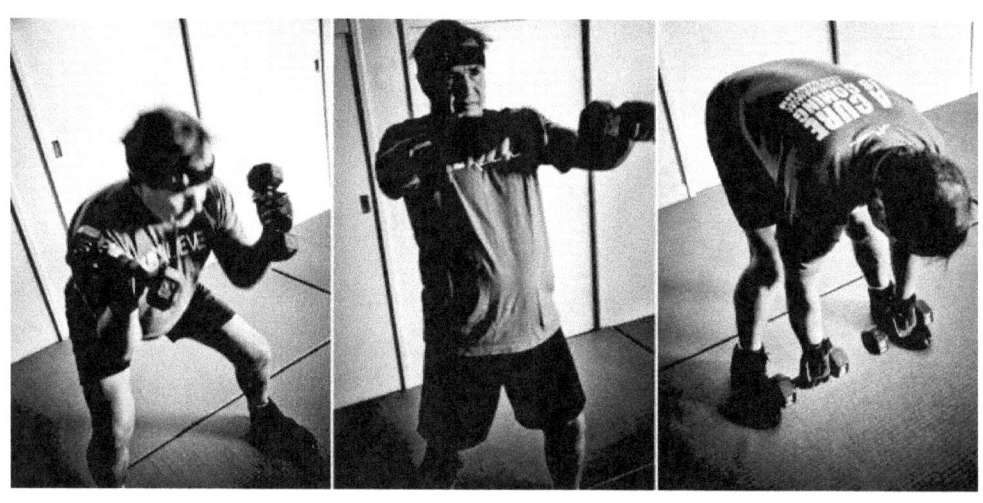

Whether you train at another gym or at mine isn't really the point.

Do you see results that last and are you really happy with yourself?

Are you making healthy decisions physically and mentally?

Are your habits aiding you or hurting you?

Find a gym that will look out for you!

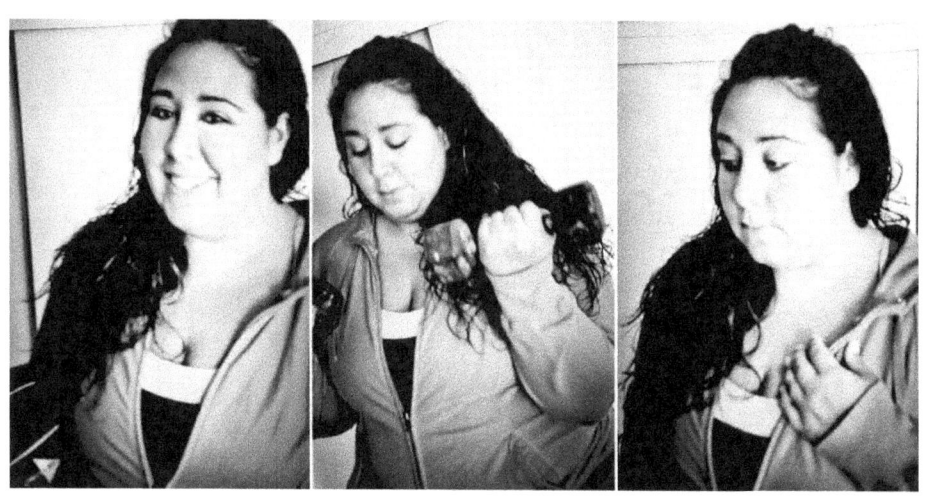

Get rid of flabby legs

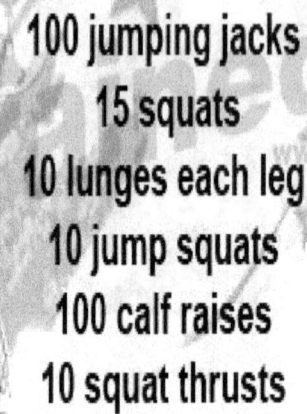

100 jumping jacks
15 squats
10 lunges each leg
10 jump squats
100 calf raises
10 squat thrusts

100 stretch kicks
100 front kicks
100 roundhouse kicks
100 side kicks
100 back kicks

theLifeSenSei.trainerze.com for the videos to exercises

You do not have to be wealthy to train, eat, or think the right way. You do not have to even train at a gym to see appreciable results. You do have to be disciplined, focused and want the best for yourself. If you have a game plan, and follow it, you will naturally succeed. If you stare at the scale and worry about the clothes that do not fit, mentally you will not overcome. You cannot listen to other people about the way you look. If you miss a session, you must start all over knowing that you do not want to settle; because you are worth it.

It is time for you to think like a rich person and be rich starting from the inside and out. You do not have to be rich to eat right, just shop smarter. Spend time at the health market instead of the grocery store. An orange instead of orange juice, bananas instead of banana pudding, wheat bread instead of white bread; healthy eating makes an enormous difference. Drink water instead of soda, fruit juice, alcohol and energy drinks. Train smart, value what you pay for; get the best trainer you can afford. Listen actively and learn the best practices that they have to offer. Better yet, train once or twice a week and copy the workout. Ask them for their advice and opinion and implement it. Think positively and before you know it, you will find your life more abundant, more enriching and plentiful; that is what being rich is to me.

Fact: America is becoming more overweight and obese

Some of you will fall into the trap of purchasing a new diet or weight loss product each year for the rest of your life. From workout videos, to abdominal machines, and to pills, you will kick, shake and crunch your way into oblivion at your homes; and that is cool. How many basement workouts lead to injury, at home workouts where the improper technique discourages results? Worse, you become addicted to overtraining and developing harmful habits. Others will sabotage themselves eating whatever they want, and putting "promise product" nonsense into their bodies. Fitness DVD's can't coach you, tweak bad habits, or challenge you after a while. You end up with a catalogue of videos that your body has gotten bored with.

When I do a complete "realistic" body analysis, I am surprised to hear so many unrealistic goals. The body analysis is not easy; it will challenge you to be honest with yourself. This lets me know if you are willing to do what it takes to see results. I measure you, weigh you and track the progress monthly. I take photos to track progress, and we realistically talk about your habits, to ensure we are both on the same page. At first my clients think I am crazy, but when they start to see the results, they love me for it. The goal is to make you fit for life not to help you just fit in some dress or suit. I have learned over the years that we are all naturally lazy and proud of our laziness. We shut off parts of the brain that want more and learn to want less. Our bodies fluctuate in shape throughout the course of our lives and we do not like ourselves because of it.

The Truth about Dieting

Dieting is the practice of eating food in a regulated fashion to achieve or maintain a controlled weight.

I'm sorry; I'm confused let's look at that again.

Definition of Diet

A: food and drink regularly provided or consumed

B: habitual nourishment

C: the kind and amount of food prescribed for a person or animal for a special reason

D: a regimen of eating and drinking sparingly so as to reduce one's weight <going on a diet>

That sounds strangely like eating to me. Ok, we need a new word to define what we are supposed to be doing in the first place. Eating in a regulated fashion is what we are supposed to be doing. Controlling our weight is what we are supposed to be doing. Alas, there lies the problem; we are not eating right or controlling our weight properly, thus, the need for dieting.

You are looking for a shortcut to achieve something you can't do normally. That shortcut is a temporary reprieve from…you. That's why you have to keep on dieting. They should make a new word for that. **Habitually dieting, chronic dieting, insanity dieting**. It is saddening to think that so many people are unfit, uncomfortable in their bodies. Though they don't seem to realize that they are the culprit and instead they complain, wish, and torment themselves while they eat unregulated. First, they let their weight get out of control; they then want to do something about it. So they try diet after diet, tip after tip, without success. **The problem isn't the dieting the problem is our habits!** Let's be honest, dieting is a tough process. Mainly, because it is a habit that you are not accustomed to. It is a process that is dreadful and not easily duplicable.

- Protein Diets, Low Fat Diets, Low Carb Diets
- Soup + Salad Diets, Specific Food + Vegetarian Diets
- Low Calorie Diets, Detox Diets
- Spray Dieting, Hormone Dieting, Fasting

How about we just eat in a regulated fashion to achieve or maintain our desired weight ALL THE TIME!

It is madness to do the same thing again and again and expect different results. You try all of these diets to no avail. While your backside gains and lose weight producing stretch marks. Your arms lose muscle definition and develop fat deposits. Cellulite forms all over your body and you cannot get rid of it because you are not working out. You should not trust yourself to know how to work out right; you cannot even trust yourself to eat right. As soon as you hear a new "diet", "fitness class", miracle process, you jump at the chance to help prove that we have become a short sighted, short cut society.

"Terence, you are being extremely tough right now. Terence you do not understand I work hard, I am so busy, my life is chaotic." No, I get it. The question is: are you getting it? When you are done "feeling" sorry for yourself, "expecting" something for nothing, "reality" should set in. Now is the time to do something about your situation. Your body is like a train, going up and down, and round and round.

When the route ends, the train gets replaced for parts if it is damaged. When you go to sleep, your body stores fat and the train is still working. It consumes energy which helps it go uphill and travel at fast speeds. You may be carrying a lot of weight, are you going uphill and traveling at fast speeds? Your body parts have mileage on them, which is why your body begins to change, regardless if you eat well and work out consistently.

Which brings us to this stunning conclusion: you have or will eventually become overweight or obese if you think working out is an option!

Here are some facts from Obesity in America.org: Obesity by the Numbers

- Obesity is the second leading cause of preventable death in the U.S.
- Approximately 127 million adults in the U.S. are overweight, 60 million are obese
- Currently, an estimated 65.2 percent of U.S. adults, age 20 years and older, and 15 percent of children and adolescents are overweight and 30.5 percent are obese.
- Approximately 62 percent of female Americans are considered overweight.
- Approximately 67 percent of male Americans are considered overweight.
- An estimated 400,000 deaths per year may be attributable to poor eating and low physical activity
- It is estimated that 25-70 percent of the difference in weight between individuals is hereditary or genetic. However, it is important to remember that genetic predisposition only impacts an individual's tendency towards obesity.
- Researchers at the U.S. Centers for Disease Control and Prevention estimated that as many as 47 million Americans may exhibit a cluster of medical conditions (a "metabolic syndrome") characterized by insulin resistance and the presence of obesity, excessive abdominal fat, high blood sugars, high blood pressure (hypertension) and high cholesterol.

There are many factors which lead to gaining weight.

- Genetics
- Abuse and Neglect
- Eating habits
- Lack of exercise

I remember what it was like to wake up every day and realize that the body I saw was not mine. I can relate knowing what it feels like to be made fun of because of my weight. Many overweight people wish they could be invisible when outside. When some TV shows inspiring weight-loss are on one channel, and another channel makes fun of larger people, I know this gives mixed messages and can be discouraging.

Maybe you were born with a little extra weight and have had a hard time losing it. Being made fun of by your peers has to take a toll on you. Maybe you gained more weight after a family member passed away or after a break up. Maybe as you got older your shape isn't what it used to be. Maybe you settled into your marriage, had children, or got into a serious accident. Whatever the reason, it's time to make a change.

The reality is if you want to make a change realistically and successfully that change has to be done a little at a time. You are going to have an uphill battle, but there is no reason why you can't win if you try your best. Most books tell you all about the problem without the solution, and ask you to take steps that may be too fast or big for you. It is already common knowledge (or is it?) with such large increases in the numbers of overweight and obese people, that the American government is concerned.

The Life Sensei says "Think about it"

It is not my place to determine who is overweight and obese; it is my job to help people become comfortable in their bodies.

Healthy People 2020 Summary of Objectives

Nutrition and Weight Status / Healthier Food Access

State nutrition standards for child care

Nutritious foods and beverages offered outside of school meals

Retail access to foods recommended by Dietary Guidelines for Americans

Health Care and Worksite Settings

Physician office visits with nutrition or weight counseling or education

Worksite nutrition and weight management classes and counseling

Weight Status

Healthy weight in adults /Obesity in adults /Obesity in children

Inappropriate weight gain

Food insecurity among households

Food and Nutrient Consumption

Fruit intake / Vegetable intake / Whole grain intake /Solid fat and added

Sugar intake /Saturated fat intake /Sodium intake /Calcium intake /

The Life Sensei says "Think about it"

America is obese; many people will get sick or die because they weigh more than they should. If you or someone you know is obese, consult your physician and fitness professional before you harm your body further. Stop cheating yourself and take control of your body.

Your Best Butt

A squats
half way down squats
full squats
cross lunges
half way down lunges
full lunges
jump squats
jump lunges
10 each
repeat for 3 min
work up to 5 mins daily

theLifeSenSei.trainerze.com for the videos to exercises

The couch potato (or get off your butt!)

When you are injured, you immediately begin to realize how much you miss being active. If you were injured in any way, you realize you cannot wait to get better. Celebrities, athletes and the average person are recognized for overcoming some type of injury and achieving success in some way. Many people, after an accident or injury have gone on to become exceptional athletes, in sports they took up after they were injured. Why were they able to overcome their injury and not only compete, but do it at a competitive, successful level?

As you get comfortable sitting on your couch after a long day of work, your body begins to shut down and your ability to get up off the couch begins to dwindle. This reaction is your body's way of saying you need rest, you do not have the energy to clean the dishes, throw that next load of clothes into the washer and you want someone else to walk the dog. (Although for some strange reason, you have no problem getting up for more dessert). Eventually, you do have to get off your butt, and this is what I want you to think about:

How do you get up off of the couch?

a) Do you have to grab something to help you up?
b) Does your stomach or back hurt when you get up?
c) Are you exerting a lot of energy while you are getting up?
d) Are you using the proper muscles while getting up?

The Life Sensei says "Think about it"

The main reason most people do not work out is because they can't move their bodies the way they would like to.

If that was too easy for you here is another test:

Lie down on the floor and stand up without using your hands or crossing your feet. Ask the same questions including these:

a) How long does it take for you to get up, did you break a sweat?
b) Do you need your hands to help you get up?
c) What muscles are you using to get up?
d) How many times can you lie down and get back up in a minute?

It seems simple on paper right? Moving your weight around is more difficult than you think. We have to be in it together, remember to find a partner who can motivate you to get outside and become more active.

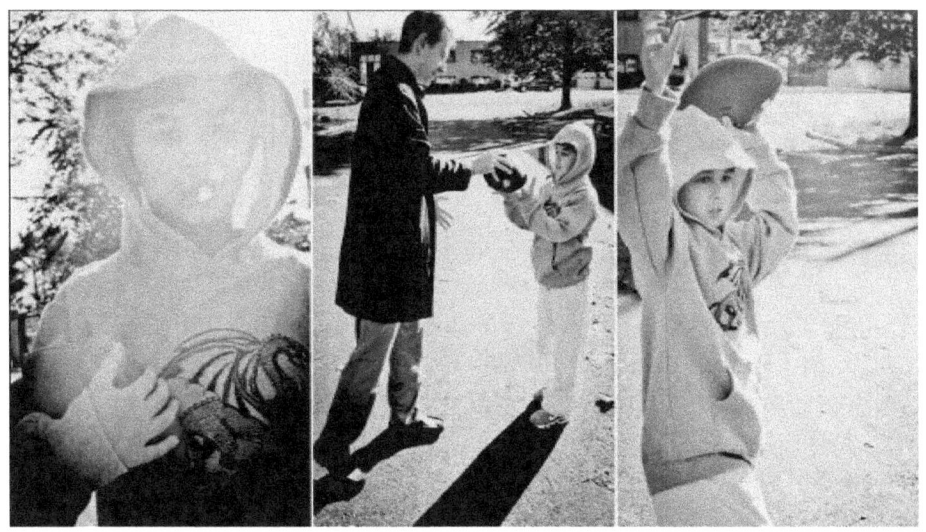

Trained 2 B Tips:

If you are willing to put in the hard work, your body will work hard for you!

It's time to get off of your butt and here are some options:

1. Start cleaning up your house.
2. Walk around your house, complex, street, local park.
3. Jog with a friend. Alternate between walking and jogging.
4. Run for a little then speed walk, run for five minutes, and then increase each week.
5. Run for 20 minutes or more.
6. Stretch by standing up and reaching for your toes hold for as long as you can.
7. Keep your legs fully extended touch your toes while you sit on your backside.
8. Use water bottles as handheld weights. Increase the size of the container for more resistance. Example: gallon of water.
9. Use basic house hold material as weights.
10. See how many pushups you can do in a minute. As you get stronger, go to 3 minutes.
11. See how many sit-ups or crunches you can do in a minute. Work your way up to 3 minutes.
12. See how many jumping jacks you can do in 3 min.
13. See how many times you can throw out alternating punches with your hands in a minute.
14. See how many times you can throw out alternating kicks with your feet in 3 minutes.
15. See how long it takes you to do all of these things (starting from #'s 10 to 14). Improve your time monthly.
16. Remember to take your time and do not force anything; go to your comfort level.
17. Enjoy the process, relax, and make sure you are consistent.

If those drills/exercises are too simple for you:

1. Clean up your house or backyard in a certain amount of time.
2. Walk or jog for a mile. Work your way up to 3 miles (track your time).
3. Run with a friend. Push each other alternating days, work up to doing it daily.
4. Sprint as fast as you can. Catch your breath then sprint again. Start with three minutes total.
5. Run for 30 minutes or more.
6. Stretch for at least 10 minutes after doing a cardio routine.
7. Use handheld weights and increase the size of weights for more resistance. Example: 2.5lbs. to 5 lbs. to 8 lbs. to 10 lbs.
8. Use barbells to do bend over rows, squats and standing toe touches.
9. See how many pushups/reverse pushups you can do in a min. Build up to sets of 10.
10. See how many sit-ups (with knees into chest) or crunches (touching your toes) you can do in a minute. Work your way up to 3 minutes.
11. See how many jumping jacks you can do or try jumping rope for 3 minutes. Increase time as you get stronger.
12. See how many times you can throw out alternating punches, changing height and tempo in five minutes.
13. See how many times you can throw out alternating kicks changing height and tempo with your feet in 5 minutes.
14. Complete entire routine in less than an hour. Then try to improve your time monthly.
15. Remember to take your time and do not force anything; go to your comfort level and pace yourself.
16. Enjoy the process, relax, be consistent, track progress and improve!

Home Workout Intermediate

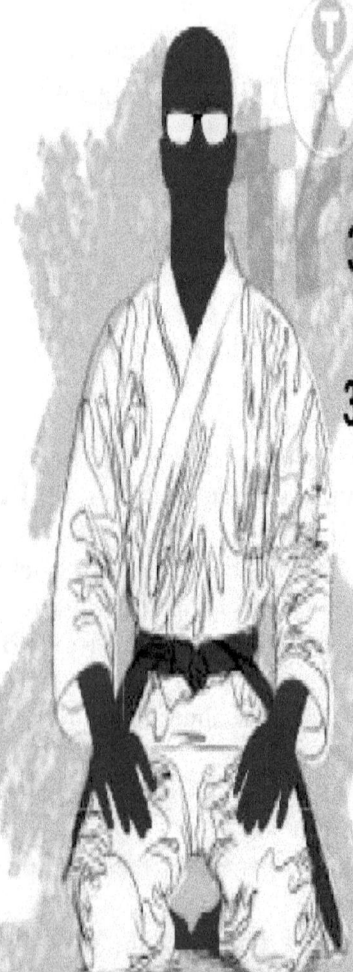

30 high knees

30 jumping jacks

30 lying leg raises

30 push ups

30 lunges each leg

30 bicycles

:30 sec plank

:30 wall squat

30 A squats

30 squat thrusts

theLifeSenSei.trainerze.com for the videos to exercises

The next thing to consider is "What are you putting into your body?" This is a touchy subject for a lot of people. There are thousands of books on dieting, eating healthy and losing weight and I'm positive that you are sick of hearing it all. Even Weight Watchers had to change their point system. So let's keep it real. You know you should be eating better, but you like what you eat. If you were better at eating you might not be reading this book to begin with, so let's not beat a dead topic, right? Here are the facts. You either are going to eat well, or you are not, so let's get straight to the point.

If you are *NOT* eating well

1. It will take a longer time to see positive results when working out.
2. Your body will have some trouble areas that will become problematic.
3. Your body will have a longer time digesting; bloating and constipation might occur.
4. You will have a slower metabolism and your body will store more fat.
5. You will have times when you feel sluggish, unmotivated and your ability to lose weight will fluctuate. You will also gain weight more easily.

If you are eating well:

1. You will see faster results if you work out consistently.
2. Your body will be leaner and healthier.
3. You will be able to go to the bathroom easier.
4. You will have a faster metabolism and your body won't store as much fat.
5. You will feel better and will be in a better position to maintain your weight or lose weight.

The Life Sensei says "think about it"

Eat for the body you want not the body you have!

If you are *NOT* eating well and are *NOT* working out

1. You will gain weight rapidly storing fat while losing muscle changing your body type in the process.
2. You will consistently become more uncomfortable with your body and develop health issues as well as possibly mental issues.
3. You will be exposed to illnesses, and injury, and become more accident prone and lethargic.
4. Your bodies will look and feel like you have done absolutely nothing and you won't be able to hide it.
5. As you gain weight your stomach muscles will expand, your blood pressure may increase and your cholesterol levels will rise.
6. Your desire to do anything physical will diminish greatly, your confidence and ability to think positively will falter. You will become comfortable with being uncomfortable in your body.

If you are eating well and working out:

1. You will see amazing results and be consistently in shape burning fat while building muscle.
2. You will have a leaner and healthier body and will have an easier time targeting problem areas.
3. Your body will be a finely tuned machine and work for you not against you.
4. You will be able to reduce your body fat intake, and will have a functional working body.
5. You will look, feel and think great. You will be able to create the body of your dreams.

The Life Sensei says "Think about it"

Set the example for your parents, family and loved ones. Take the time to educate those you care about. Realize eating healthy and living healthy is no longer an option. Change for the better together today.

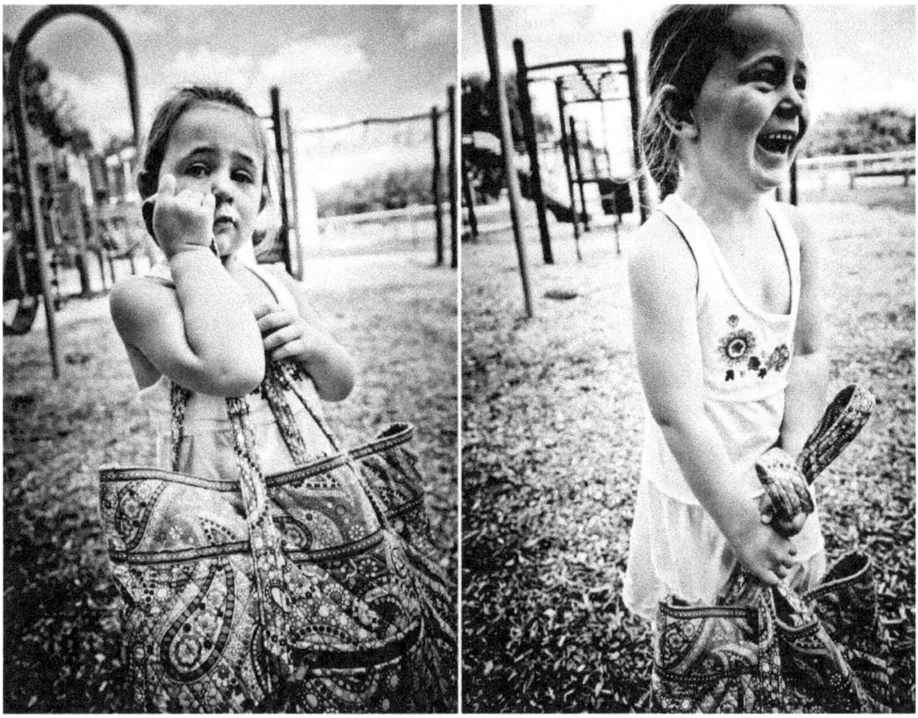

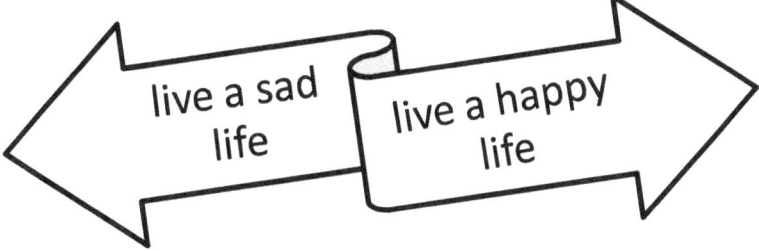

live a sad life

live a happy life

The Life Sensei on Food

For those interested in shedding excess fat, wait after finishing your cardio workout to eat. This enables your body to burn more calories during the period immediately following your cardio workout, when your heart rate remains higher than usual.

Drink plenty of water or other calorie-free beverages. People sometimes confuse thirst with hunger. So you can end up eating extra calories when an ice-cold glass of water is really what you need.

Think about what you can add to your diet, not what you should take away. Start by focusing on getting the recommended 5-9 servings of fruits and vegetables each day.

Consider whether you're really hungry. Whenever you feel like eating, look for physical signs of hunger. Hunger is your body's way of telling you that you need fuel, so when a craving doesn't come from hunger, eating will never satisfy it.

When you're done eating, you should feel better, not stuffed, bloated, or tired. Your stomach is only the size of your fist, so it takes just a handful of food to fill it comfortably.

The most common mistake most people make is not eating after they train or not eating the right thing. This meal should contain a mixture of different types of carbohydrates like glucose, maltodextrin and fructose.

Glucose will cause an insulin spike to drive the nutrients into the muscle. The maltodextrin will be used to fill up the muscles with glycogen. Fructose should be included to replenish liver glycogen that has been used during training. The post workout meal should have at least 20% of your daily protein needs.

To calculate your post workout protein needs take .20 times your body weight. (For example I would take 260 x .20 = 52 grams.)

What are you spending your money on? Are you seeing results, and are you happy? Yes, the two should go hand-in-hand although they may not do so all the time. Value your time and energy and your body will reward you.

SIMPLE: Eat often and do not exercise. Just continue to eat all the crap you know you shouldn't. Exercise is a curse word.

AVERAGE: Eat more to gain and pay less to lose. Spend an average of $60 a month for coffee, an average of $15 a month for a membership you may not use.

GREAT! : Eat less to lose weight the healthy way and play more to maintain your weight. Shop smart, eat smaller meals more consistently. Do something, anything, every day. Think like the rich to become a wealthier, healthier you.

BALANCE: Plan ahead. To enjoy the good times and weather thebad, don't get to high and don't get to low. Be prepared for the unexpected as best as you possibly can.

The Life Sensei says, "Thinks about it"

Running/jogging is a great exercise but it's not "one size fits all". Heavier runners produce more body heat which means that they can sweat more, so drinking water is important. Heavier runners also put more pressure on joints and shoes, so make sure to watch the tread thickness of shoes. Watch your joint health and speed to ensure safety and enjoyment so you can make it a life style change.

Martial guidance for life's journey

Food Journal

I have met so many people that wanted to learn to eat right. Very few of those people know about proper nutrition or were committed to following what I would like to call a life style change. When people ask me what they should eat, I first ask them for a journal of what they do eat. Keeping a journal of what you put into your body has several purposes:

- It helps you keep track of eating when you are supposed to.
- It forces you to think about what you are putting into your body.
- It lets me know if you are serious about changing your eating habits (Most people aren't initially).
- It allows you to see improvements in your eating habits as you continue.
- It serves as a reminder to your growth as a healthy individual.

Do you keep track of your bank statements? Well your body is a bank as well; be sure your deposits are healthy, smart choices if you want to see good returns on your body's investments. Diabetes, cellulite, wrinkles, fat deposits, and high cholesterol are all indicative of genetics, lifestyle and **poor eating habits.**

Start your journal right now and make it work for you

Get a notebook and start with the first day of the week, take the time to be honest and descriptive. If you can, write down what you ate and what you wanted to eat as well. Take the time to fill this out right after you eat. Make sure you add snacks also. For the great minded fill it out before and commit to the meal. If you follow this for a month your diet will change simply because you'll be watching what you eat. With proper coaching and health tips you should start to see a change in the way your body looks in a little more than a few months. If you have an eating disorder or will go insane with a journal put it on your refrigerator instead and try to keep it light with a positive attitude.

Burn 100+ calories Now!

March in place
Jog in place
Jumping Jacks
Long Jumps
Jog Lightly
Jumping Jacks
Squat and Kick, Alternate Legs
Jog lightly
Long Jumps

Each exercise for 1 minute

theLifeSenSei.trainerze.com for the videos to exercises

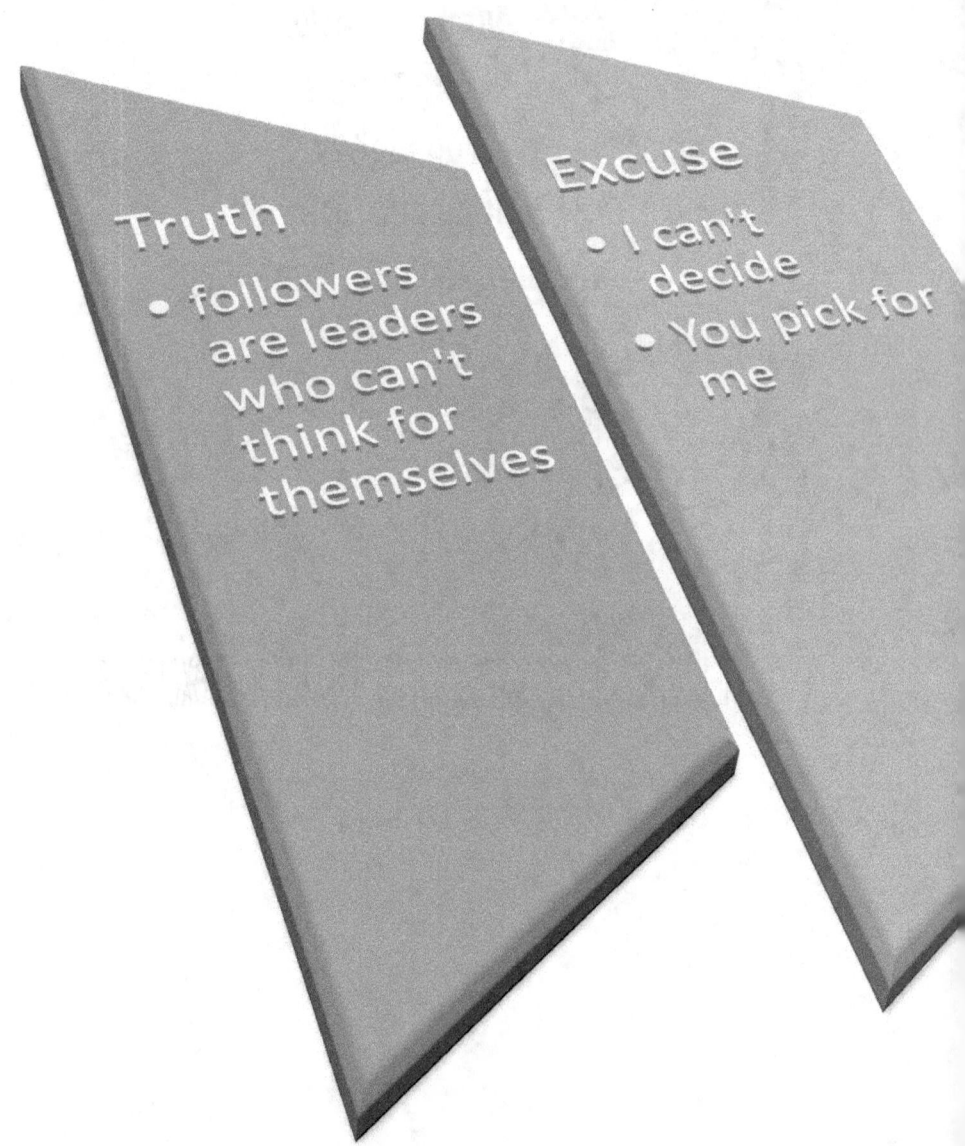

Truth
- followers are leaders who can't think for themselves

Excuse
- I can't decide
- You pick for me

Plan

Make sure your Doc is knowledgeable ask questions

Mention triglycerides, HDL/LDL ratio

Your diet + exercise habits can eliminate the need for drugs

Do not be afraid to eat fat it is still necessary for your body

Implement

Make time work for you and combine

Cardio, Strength Training, Core + Skill exercises in 1 workout!

Be open-minded + learn a martial art

A humble body is a strong body

Habit

Plan Ahead

If you can't visualize it do not do it

"Fake it until you make it" **Michelle Buenafuente Phillips**

Desire more for yourself + Desire the Best

Results

Sleep (enough said)

6 to 8 hours / 20 min power nap

5th Stop: *Visual Aid*

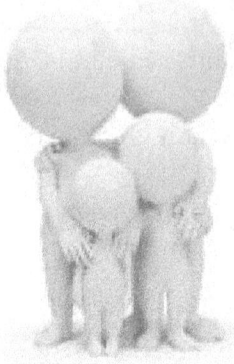

Do fit people have a better life? Yes!

Fewer heart attacks + health issues

Non smokers less chances of getting cancer

Less chances of injuries + getting colds

More money + reduced medical expenses

Live a longer, prosperous life!

Focus on the skill sets from the Trained 2 B chapter. Work on yourself first and then share with your friends and loved ones. This will rub off on everyone you meet, making work and play enjoyable, making you happier and helping you get in the best shape you can personally be in.

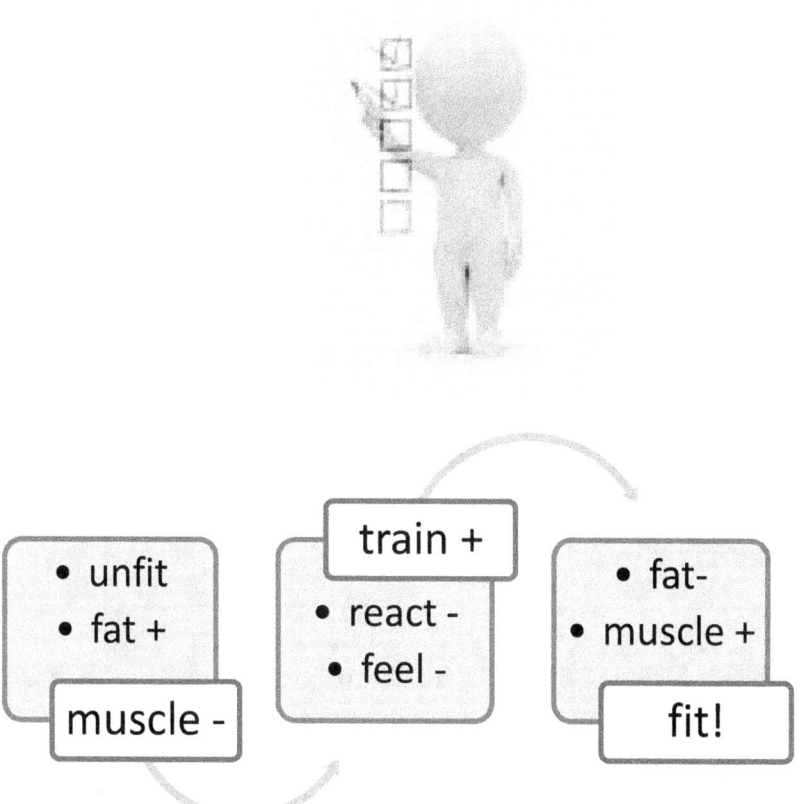

A person who is fit will have an easier time getting rid of fat. Getting out of shape and suffering muscle loss makes you lose the ability to get rid of fat. Fat controls how you feel about your body and how it reacts. Muscle is important because it demands every part of the body to work harder. The more muscle you use, the less you have to work out. The Trained System knows that working out to get fit is not the same as working out to lose fat.

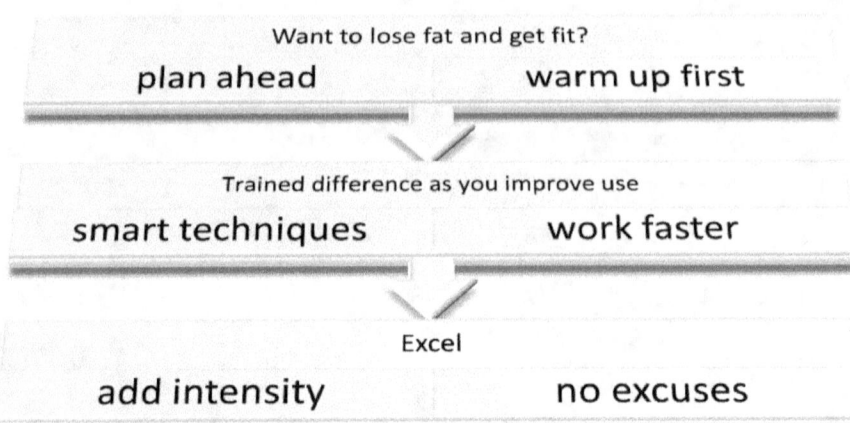

Want to lose fat and get fit?

plan ahead	warm up first

Trained difference as you improve use

smart techniques	work faster

Excel

add intensity	no excuses

Losing muscle reduces your ability to burn calories and regulate your blood sugar, it also makes you weaker. Lost muscle is also replaced by fat when you stop dieting, making your skin look as if you have more flabby areas. Remember, each pound of fat takes up 18 percent more space on your body than each pound of muscle. Realistically, different people lose weight without losing muscle the healthiest way when they lose:

Obese to morbidly obese: 3 to 5 pounds per week

Overweight: 2 to 3 pounds per week

Lean to average: 1 to 2 pounds per week

Very Lean: 0.5 to 1 pound per week

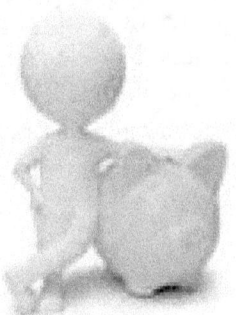

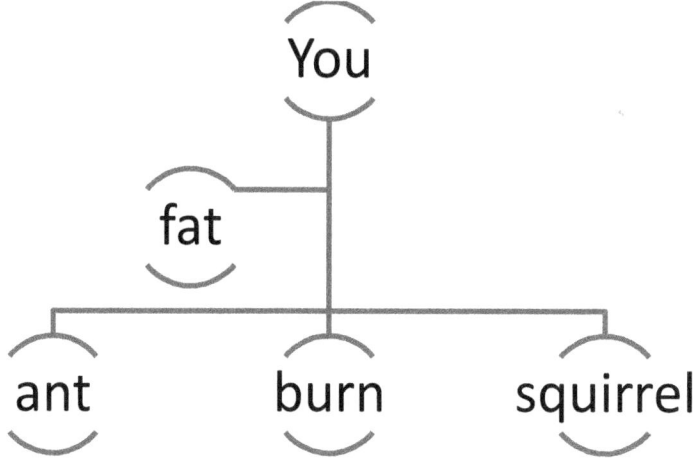

Every personal training client gets the ant and squirrel speech, in relation to how fat is stored and burned. The ant stores fat for energy and the squirrel stores fat for storage. When you exercise you want to use the fat for storage to burn and lose weight, while using the fat for energy to maximize your workouts. At the same time, the ant and squirrel are going to fight you; neither wants to give up what they stored. You need to build a consistent relationship to let the ant and squirrel know they can trust you. Replace the energy with healthy foods while working out so that your body won't have the desire to store fat all the time.

Then remember these tips as you start your weight loss program:

You will plateau: Weight will drop at first, meaning you'll lose a steady amount initially. As you get lighter, your weight will tend to drop slower. Don't get frustrated if weight holds for a few days, or even a couple of weeks. The closer you get to your goal, the longer your weight plateaus.

Time out: Every 8 to 12 weeks, take 5 days off eat what you like.

Redefine progress: There are other means of success besides the scale. Monitor your triglycerides, blood pressure, and body fat percentage. As these numbers improve, you'll have even more motivation to stick with your fitness goals.

Your body produces energy three ways.

creatine

lactate

aerobic

Only one of them burns fat.

Creatine phosphate doesn't need oxygen, fat or sugar to function. Energy lasts naturally for about ten seconds, that's why athletes use creatine products. It's not the lack of these or pain from lactic acid that makes you stop working out, it's running out of creatine. Think about sprints, plyometric and intense workouts as examples.

Lactate burns sugar, oxygen isn't needed. Think of the workouts as more than a sprint and less than running a mile. Like an in-between work out, energy lasts naturally for about six to eight minutes. You run out of sugar quick and build lactic acid. The trick is to get more sugar into your muscle while ridding it of lactate.

Aerobic burns sugar and fat, however, oxygen is needed and gives infinite energy. Think of a marathon, one lb. of fat = 3,500 calories of energy. Aerobic exercise describes systemic exercise, which improves the health of the whole body. Want to lose fat when you work out? Mix up your workouts so that you maximize the three different ways to use energy.

Make it happen!

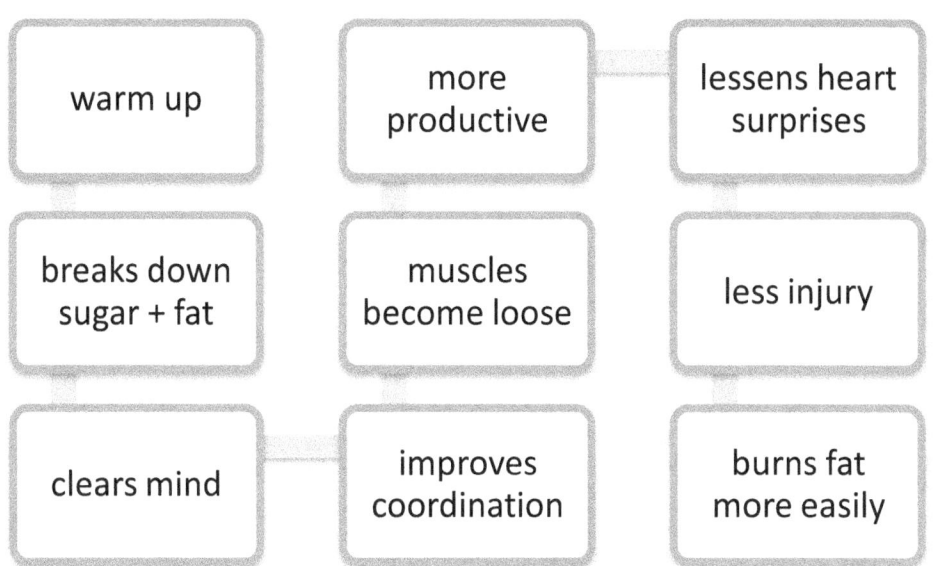

A good idea for a warm up is doing a slower version of your workout. Some form of aerobic exercise, including jumping jacks or jogging in place.

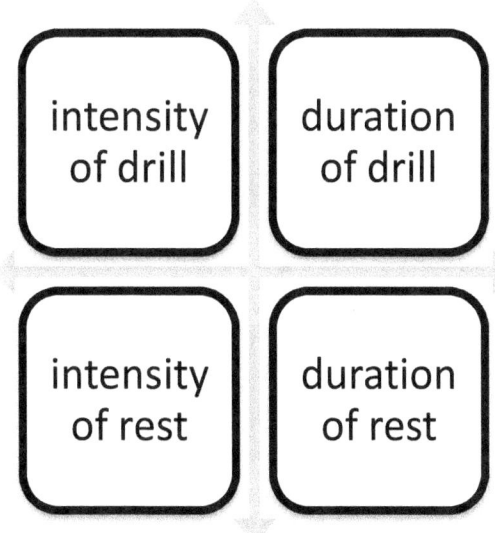

What are my workouts known for? Pushing you to your breaking point to achieve maximum results and making sure you are smiling while you do it!

If training intensely for short period drills or long periods breathe properly and catch your breath before moving to next drill.

If training in-between or stop and go drills, you should not catch your breath completely.

Remember if you exercise too much it's the same as too little.

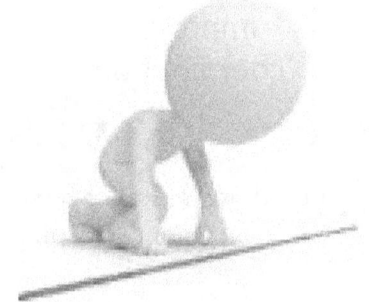

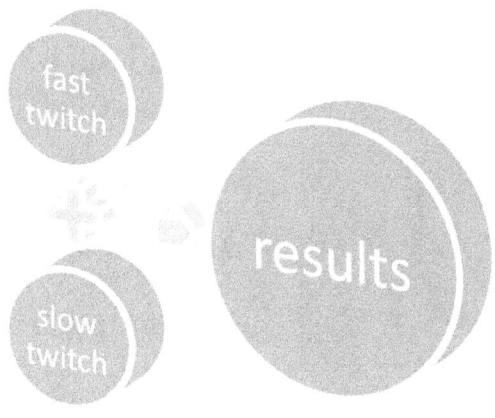

Fast twitch muscles are sugar burners, quick and strong. They contract fast and forcefully. You will like these because they will enhance the shape of your muscles. They also protect against injury but build up lactic acid quickly.

Slow twitch muscles are fat burners, needed for endurance. They contract slowly and with less force. They do most of the difficult work, like aerobics for example. Fast twitch muscles jump in to help when necessary. They can get fuel from sugar or lactic acid.

TRUTH

These visual aids should help you when you need to see what you are trying to accomplish. They should motivate and inspire you to dream, set goals and commit to them.

the LifeSensei Workout Challenge

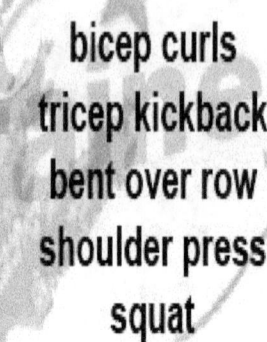

bicep curls
tricep kickback
bent over row
shoulder press
squat

:30 jumping lunges
:30 plank
:30 bicycles
in between each weight drill

theLifeSenSei.trainerze.com for the videos to exercises

Plan

If you write down different ways to make exercise fun

You will achieve results while your fat runs

Spend more days enjoying the sun

Implement

Body Analysis

You need to accept your body for what it is

Realistically learn what shape your body is + how to train it

Get over old image and create new image

Habit

PMS info! Men need to know this too

Women want more carbs when their estrogen levels drop

2 weeks before her period decreasing her mood-lifting hormones

This motivates eating fat + calorie rich snacks

Support the special women in your life

Results

Abdominals they do not get tired, neither should you

Train Them Daily, Rest 1 Day

The Life Sensei on "Mood/Food" relationships

Food is important; skip regular meals and exercise and we feel tired and cranky. When we go too long without eating, our blood sugar crashes and mood swings begin. This leads to reaching for caffeine and sugar to temporarily feel better, which is followed by a crash and the cycle, repeats itself. More stress leads to sleeping less so we wake up feeling tired and cranky.

Caffeine can enhance physical and mental performance, but too much can spur anxiety and nervousness. In terms of feeling better or having more energy, it's better to drink water. Dairy products contain whey protein, which alleviates stress, improves mood, and enhances memory giving a sense of relaxation. If you're not a milk person, green tea fights depression and helps combat stress.

If we don't eat any carbohydrates we are likely going to feel tired, angry, and depressed. Simple carbohydrates bring our mood down. Complex carbohydrates have a positive effect on mood. Our body needs carbohydrates to produce serotonin a chemical that elevates mood, suppresses appetite, and has a calming effect also playing a role in sleep. Combining carbohydrates and proteins enhances the availability of serotonin in your brain.

Low omega-3 levels are associated with depression, negative outlooks and rash thinking. Omega-3s improve both mood and memory.

Getting enough iron increases sociability, and your overall energy level. Not enough iron in your system leads to depression, inactivity, fatigue, and decreased self-confidence.

High saturated fats are linked to sluggishness, depression and dementia. Our bodies take a while to digest fat and the process leaves you feeling empty. This means that you have to develop sound strategies to prevent your food dictating how you will behave. If you eat healthier you will be a better person inside and out.

Martial guidance for life's journey

When writing out your goals remember to include a timetable to complete goals, a realistic schedule, a fall back plan, a punishment for not sticking to your goals, and make sure you have some fun.

Writing Out Your Goals

1. Grab a pen or pencil (and an eraser in case you decide to change your mind).
2. Grab a piece of paper; preferably a notebook that you can use solely for your goal setting.
3. Find a quiet place to write down your thoughts.
4. Break down the order of importance.
5. Take a look at the thoughts and make goals to your satisfaction.
6. Walk away from your notebook and come back in five minutes.
7. If your goals still make sense begin to look for your training partner.

Writing Out Your Goals with your Training Partner

1. Grab a pencil (definitely bring an eraser).
2. Open up your notebook, and if you really like your partner hand them a notebook.
3. Find a quiet place to go over your hopes and dreams; share your goals.
4. Write down common goals and make plans to complete them.
5. Take a look at each other's goals and make sure they are realistic.
6. Walk away from goal setting, have a cup of tea, go see a movie or better yet start training.
7. Begin to implement your goals immediately.

If you do not write out your goals you may still be able to complete some of your hopes and dreams. Most people will need to write down the goals to remember them. So write them down already!

Crunches Bicycles & Planks

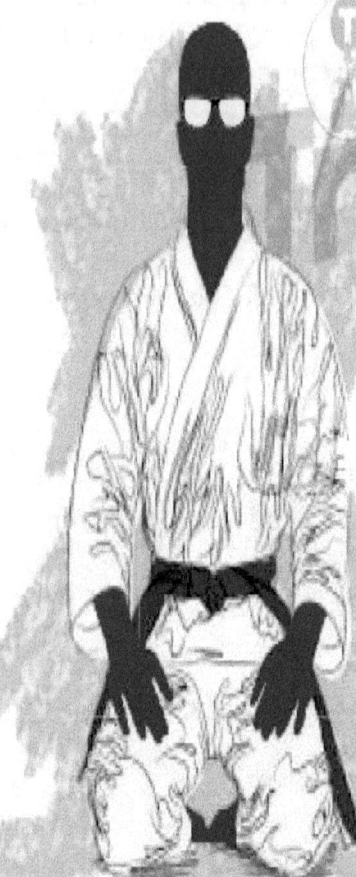

10 crunches

15 bicycles

:30 sec plank

:20 sec plank

10 crunches

20 bicycles

:20 sec plank

10 crunches

:30 sec plank

30 bicycles

theLifeSenSei.trainerze.com for the videos to exercises

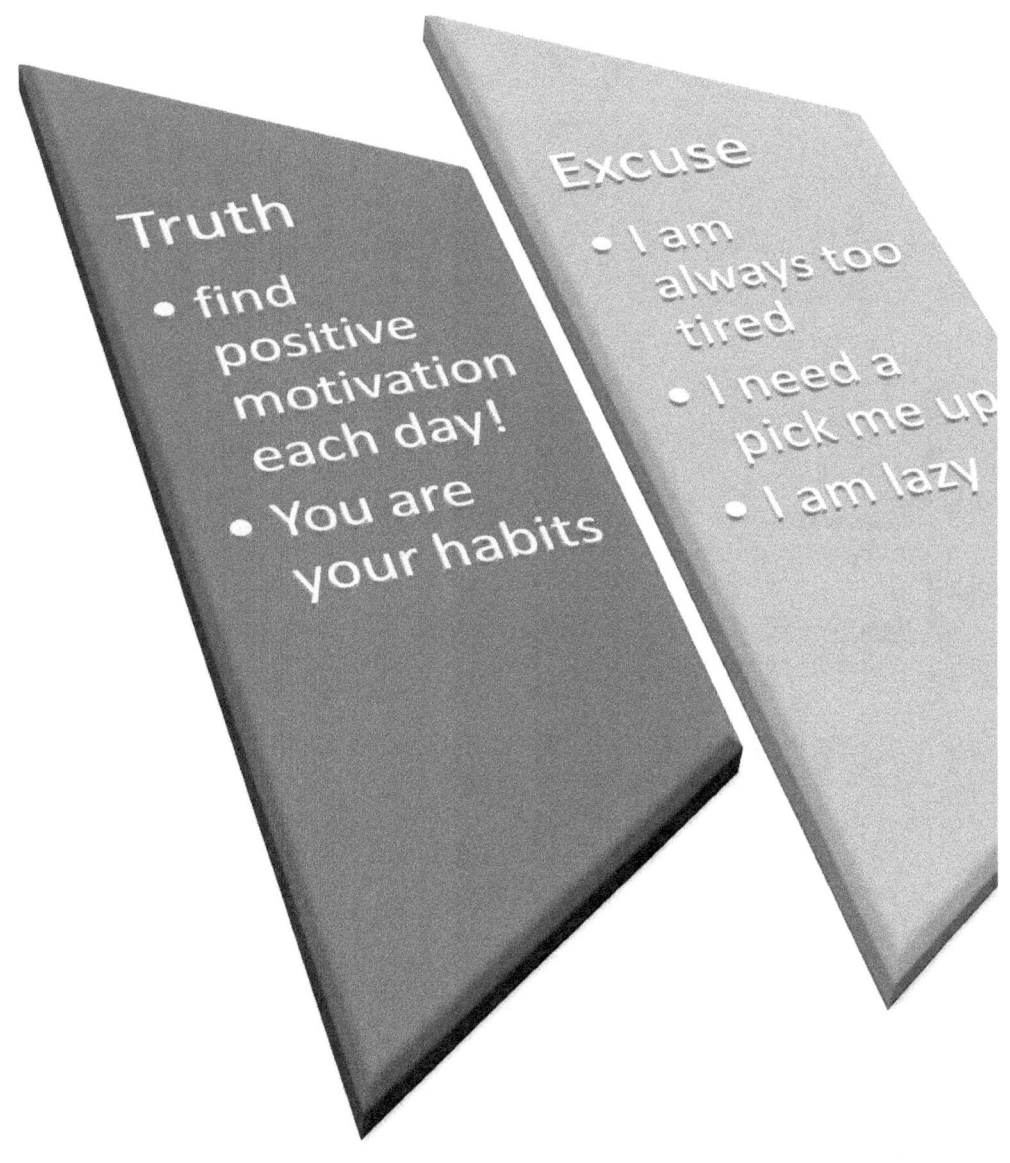

Truth
- find positive motivation each day!
- You are your habits

Excuse
- I am always too tired
- I need a pick me up
- I am lazy

Final Stop: *Trained Healthy Mindset*

The Trained Mindset

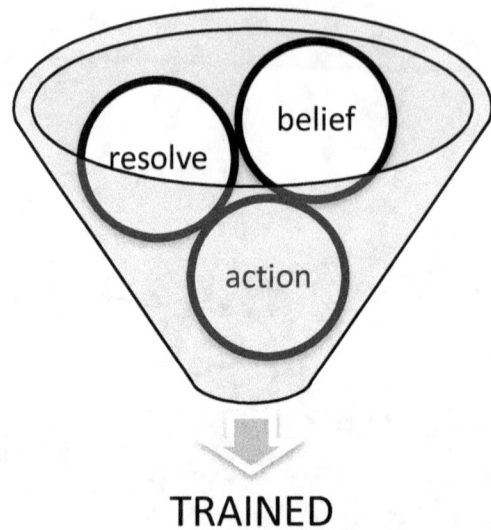

TRAINED

<u>Belief</u>: Know what you believe in and build a strong foundation that you can depend on.

<u>Resolve</u>: Find a solution to any problem you have; make a decision and stick with it.

<u>Action</u>: Achieve your purpose; do not stop until you reach your goals. Then set new goals.

<u>Train</u>: Learn the skills necessary to do a job, especially through practical experience. Improve something, especially the mind with discipline.

1. Put in the hard work. Be dedicated.
2. Never take a day off. Work mentally, spiritually, physically and/or emotionally.
3. Excuses are excuses. Save the sorry for when you really mean it.
4. Accept the way you feel about something and separate it from what you expect and the way something is.
5. Life rewards those who live it.
6. Develop skill sets that will benefit you in multiple ways.
7. Put your Faith in GOD. (Most importantly trust your beliefs in your Higher Power.)

Every time I have a moment of weakness, I think about my students, friends, loved ones, or those less fortunate in life and realize I'm going to be fine. I get a hold of my negative feelings and put it in a choke hold. I grit my teeth, place a firm grip on my dreams and put it into action. That is what a fighter does, what someone who cares does for themselves and others. I think about the investments I made when starting to work out and train. I think about the students who quit or the clients that stop exercising and know they will regret it. I smile when I hear that my philosophy and school are different from the rest. I am happy that these principles touch so many lives.

The Life Sensei says, "Think about it"

Set a goal, make sure it is realistic and in your best interest and then get it done.

The Machine

After your goals are set, you begin your mission. It may take a while before it bears fruits. If you allow yourself to become complacent, your mission can be aborted. You must become a machine, programmed to operate and fulfill its duty, no excuses. Without feelings, machines perform to the level they were designed for at an optimum amount of years. Machines do what needs to get done, period. When you press play, it starts. When you press stop, it ends. When you press pause, it doesn't fast forward, it pauses. It doesn't ask you what you mean when performing a task, nor does it second guess itself. It simply does what it was meant to do. When a machine gets old or obsolete it is repaired, replaced or destroyed.

Similarly the Trained Mindset gets you to think and perform like a machine. Program yourself, operate and fulfill your duty to yourself, your family, your friends and community, no excuses. Your body cannot be destroyed so you have to consistently upgrade it yourself. You must train your mind to accomplish whatever it sets itself to do. Do not let feelings cloud your judgment or delay your mission. Fulfill your role like a machine and see your desires and dreams come true.

Home Workout Advance

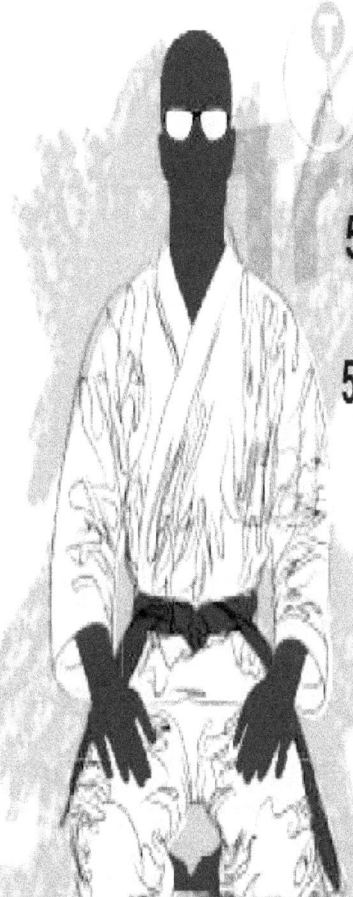

50 high knees
50 jumping jacks
50 lying leg raises
50 push ups
50 lunges each leg
50 bicycles
:60 sec plank
:60 wall squat
50 A squats
50 squat thrusts

theLifeSenSei.trainerze.com for the videos to exercises

Excuses versus the Truth

Excuse: there are more things important than my health.

Truth: Yes, there are more important things than your health. Your faith, your motives and how you treat others.   The legacy you leave behind and how you love others. All of those things are predicated on your health. How healthy you are will dictate what you do with your life, how you impact others with the opportunities given, and the lessons you share as a result of your experiences.

Excuse: My ideal weight was when I was younger, or before I had kids.

Truth: If you're hoping to get back to what you weighed a few years ago, I would back you on that. However, if you're looking at 10 or more years your expectations are not realistic. Many people put on weight as they get older, and a slower metabolism makes it harder to lose weight and change your body as easily as you did when you were younger. Don't live in the past! Set a goal that works for the way you live now.

Excuse: This is too difficult for me.

Truth: It is difficult for everyone; you will not be the first or the last person to experience this feeling. You can however, be the next person to help change that perspective. As we speak there are thousands of other people making the decision to make it work.

Excuse: My ideal weight belongs on a standard height and weight chart.

Truth: Many factors play a role in determining your weight, such as your body type, the number of fat cells you have, and how muscular you are. The numbers on a standard body mass index (BMI) chart are just approximations, and may not be the best gauge of good health. Studies show they may under-count some women as overweight by not measuring body fat and over-count others who have a higher ratio of muscle to fat. Chart your expectations with reality and the way you look and feel.

Excuse: I'm comfortable with the way I am.

Truth: I will agree with you on one point. You "believe that you are comfortable"; behind that belief is a gnawing feeling of you wanting to change, evolve and be better. Listen to that feeling, it is the beginning of an expectation for you to change, evolve and be better. Depending on what you do it will become either a reality or remain a belief.

Excuse: My ideal weight is the lowest number I've hit on past diets.

Truth: The fact that you're dieting means that you've gained some, if not all, of your old weight back. If you set a weight-loss goal or program that's not realistic, you'll fail in an unhealthy cycle of yo-yo dieting. Such repeated weight loss and regaining can alter your body composition, lowering the amount of muscle mass you have. This, in turn, can slow your metabolism and make those flabby arms, backside and tummy more pronounced. So what's your best weight goal? The one you can actually live with.

Excuse: It shouldn't/ doesn't matter.

Truth: To whom? You believe it doesn't matter to your peers, family, or loved ones? I am 100% positive that those who care about you will be encouraged, proud and amazed at a new healthier you. What about the haters, enemies or the general public? Who cares what the negative minded think? If you do though, wouldn't you rather have a positive impact on them?

Excuse: The less I weigh, the healthier I'll be.

Truth: Many studies show that if you're overweight, losing just 5 to 10 percent of your current weight is all you have to do to reap the bulk of the health benefits associated with weight loss: lower risk of heart disease, stroke, diabetes, and even some forms of cancer. You have to start somewhere, start with the 5 percent and renew your commitment once you have achieved your goals the right way.

Trained

Trains move from one stop to the next picking up thousands of passengers along the way. It helps people get to where they need to go so they can do what they need to do. The ride can be bumpy, but it reaches its goal consistently at an amazing percentage. If it gets derailed, it gets repaired and right back on track. It works throughout the day and night, for all seasons, without breaks or any one feeling sorry for it. It is a thankless job, but a job nonetheless.

Trained definition: 1. To develop or form the habits, thoughts, or behavior by discipline and instruction. 2. To make proficient by instruction and practice, as in some art, profession, or work. 3. To make (a person) fit by proper exercise, diet, practice, etc., as for an athletic performance. 4. To bring to bear on some object; point, aim, or direct, as a firearm, camera, fist, or eye. 5. To entice; allure.

Being trained is setting yourself up for success by simply being you. Continue to build good habits and slowly remove the bad ones. Be honest with yourself and refuse to allow excuses to get the better of you.

What are you Trained to do?

Becoming healthier require you to let go of what you think you know and open yourself up to be taught. As you begin to develop the techniques and can apply them frequently with fewer mistakes you are on your way to understanding them better. As your understanding grows, so does your awareness, confidence and ability. Then your habits begin to change, you begin to see new results and develop consistency. Your positive habits then begin to become healthy routines that before you know it become who you are and what you are about.

This becomes contagious and spreads like wildfire throughout all your endeavors, you become more successful in life, more confident. You have more opportunities to live the life you have intended and dreamed for yourself. Your family, friends and peers will follow suit, they will want to copy your success and practice what you have accomplished. Then you can use one another positively to improve upon your dreams.

The Planning mindset: you set goals throughout the day with an open mind. Being adaptable you set realistic goals and never divert from them. Even if you are distracted, you keep the eyes on the prize and stay focused. You enjoy the simple things in life without being simple-minded. Your family and loved ones know they are valued and you are committed to the happiness of others as well as yourself; because you think and plan ahead for value and happiness.

The Implementing mindset: you stay focused on conducting your affairs with a purpose-filled demeanor. Accomplishing your goals and fulfilling your commitments is your duty and purpose. You excel in your endeavors with a renewed vigor daily so you can succeed consistently. When you are finish putting your nightly dreams into your daily efforts you can move on to....

The Habit mindset: you stay mindful of all you survey; you are relaxed and tense at the same time. You long for peace even though you are prepared for war. Your decisions are thought out and calculated, weighed and measured. You are an ambassador for doing things the right way because it will produce the right results in the future. Conducting yourself with grace and humbleness, you are the example of execution and consistency. The more you continue to build beneficial exercises and drills the more it becomes a part of who you are.

The Results mindset: you see the efforts falling into place and admire your efforts for a moment and move on to the next. The world is waiting for you to conquer it and it is dependent on your every move. Your body, mind, friends and peers are waiting for you to slip so they can make excuses, You don't slip, because you have planned, built a solid mindset, forge positive practices and now enjoy the fruits of your labor. You can rest peacefully tomorrow new challenges are waiting.

The Life Sensei says "Think about it

Where you dine may affect your appetite. Areas with warmer colors will make you hungry thus causing you to eat more. Cooler color areas may make you eat up to 30% less.

Many people are these modes some of the time or at various times in their lives. I believe to be truly at your personal best you have to be mindful of these different modes all of the time. Whether you are going to the supermarket, spending time with your family, forced to defend yourself or at a conference meeting be prepared.

Knowing what you are capable of and how you would act in different situations is a valuable tool. Whether you act, react, freeze or forget is totally in your control. You learn about yourself when you work out and reach that last set or while running that last lap when you are already tired. When you learn about yourself, you can resolve your differences, resulting in better overall understanding. When you excel during the month of doom (a period where I torture my clients at the school so they can see how they have progressed) and you realize it was not that terrible after all, you realize who you have become.

When you can look in the mirror and accept yourself, when you eat properly and consistently follow healthy habits because you care you realize your self-worth. When you know you have belief, resolve and you act on it, you know that you are trained.

Trained 2 B your Personal Best

You do not know what life has in store for you, are you trained to be ready when something difficult comes your way? One day, you can be going through the rollercoaster's of life, making the most of your situation. The next day you can be forced to get off the ride. When you are faced with a life threatening illness, that rollercoaster seems like a much better option, than being forced to see everyone else get to ride.

Let's take cancer, for example. This is a general disease which has nothing general about it. It can attack the prostate, breast, and pretty much every part of your body with devastating effect. No one is immune to it; unfortunately, many lose their battle with it. We need to find a cure. My grandmother was blessed and survived. She goes out and takes fitness classes, and hangs out with her friends. She plays videogames that keep her fit and maintains a positive attitude.

What if you have a family to take care of? What if your life was complicated to begin with and then you found out you had cancer? How would you deal with that adversity? One of my clients was a kick boxing student, who had children who wanted to take Karate. For a few years, I watched this family grow and deal with life as best as they could. Eventually, this client joined Karate and was challenged yet gave 100%. This client always kept a smile, regardless of the circumstance.

When I began to look for help with this book, this person jumped at the chance to help. Previously, I was disappointed that many who wanted to help did not. I was reluctant to receive help, but, opened myself up to trusting the client who also became my friend. We began the process of working on the book, and tragedy struck.

The diagnosis was cancer.

What do you say to someone, who remains positive, and seems too often to get the short end of the stick? You do not say anything. You support them, pray for them, and aid them whenever possible. You hope for a speedy recovery knowing that you have no control.

I get many clients who are unsure whether they want to train, who sabotage their training by never letting go of their fear, and who quit before they start. This is frustrating, but a part of the job. What about the clients who want to train but cannot? This cancer-stricken client continued to come to the school for as long as possible, until it was no longer possible. They fought a battle tougher than any sparring session, harder than dealing with racism, or facing their demons. I was amazed that this client would still call, visit and try to make classes even though her body would fail her.

That is being "Trained". Not giving up on their dreams, not lying down when challenged. Not giving up, when most would say it is understandable to quit.

She is a survivor, a fighter like many before her and many after. The client still managed to be a part of the editing process. The client remains optimistic, and is an example of the **TRAINED MINDSET**. I cannot take credit for that. If it is in you then it is in you. I believe it is in all of us.

I hope that you make the most of this opportunity; this call for you to become your absolute best. What is the alternative? I began this journey unsure of where it would take me. Honestly, there are many times I do not know what the outcome will be. I will not worry; I will be true to what I believe in and fight for what I know to be right.

Life is short, but it does not have to be. You can decide to live a life that is incredible if you will give yourself a chance. You can live a fit life, a passionate life and be truly happy. There is no guarantee, no promise that it will always go your way. You will face trials and face opposition in life. The only guarantee that you can make is to yourself, that you will be able to trust and depend on you. The promise will be that you will fight until your last breath. When people see that, they will know that you have lived.

TRUTH

Live your life with a level of commitment that you can be proud of. You do not have to be the world's best. You do have to be your personal best. That is and should always be your goal. Get the most out of yourself every day.

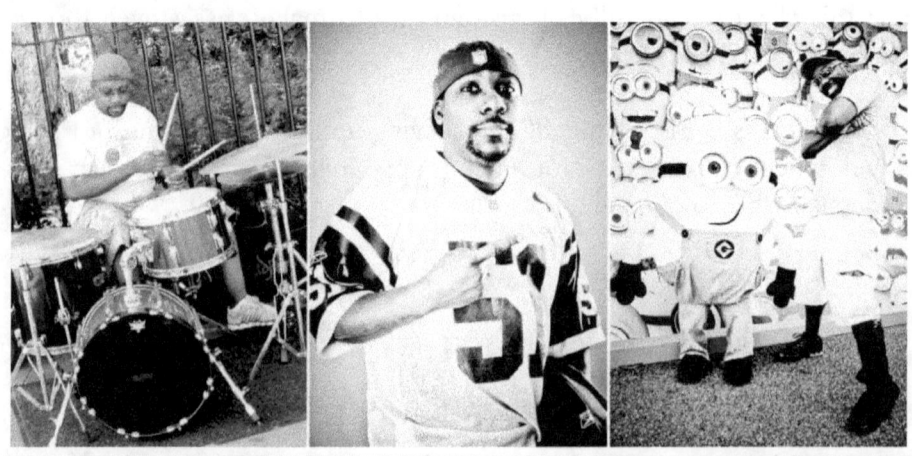

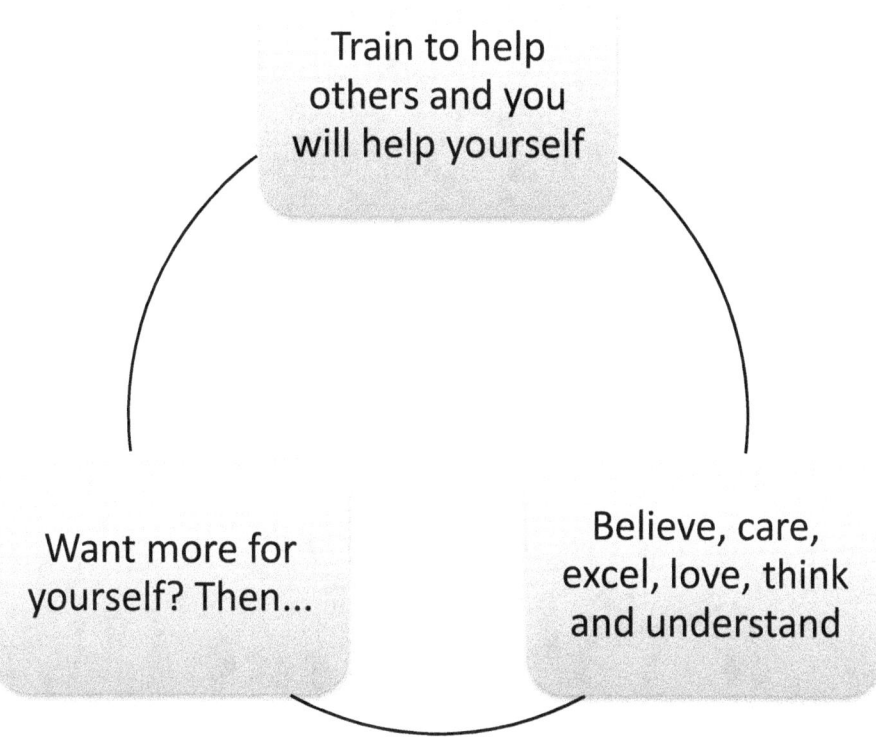

Train to help others and you will help yourself

Believe, care, excel, love, think and understand

Want more for yourself? Then...

Great! : You.

Think About it: Whatever it takes.

5-4-3-2-1 Workout

5 min

any cardio you want

4min

lunges or mountain climbers

3 min

10 push ups or 20 tricep dips

rest then repeat

2 min

:30 seconds of each

squats-squat hops

1 min

plank

theLifeSenSei.trainerze.com for the videos to exercises

The Life Sensei on Results

Never go two weeks without a change.

Train your mind, body and spirit for maximum results.

Don't get to high on yourself or too low.

Double your efforts but don't obsess.

Learn to relax and appreciate your efforts.

Treat yourself to something nice.

If the average American got 10 more minutes of sleep every working day it would add up to 40 more hours of sleep a year.

Reassess your goals every two months.

Impossible is a word means I'm possible.

Results are predicated on starting something.

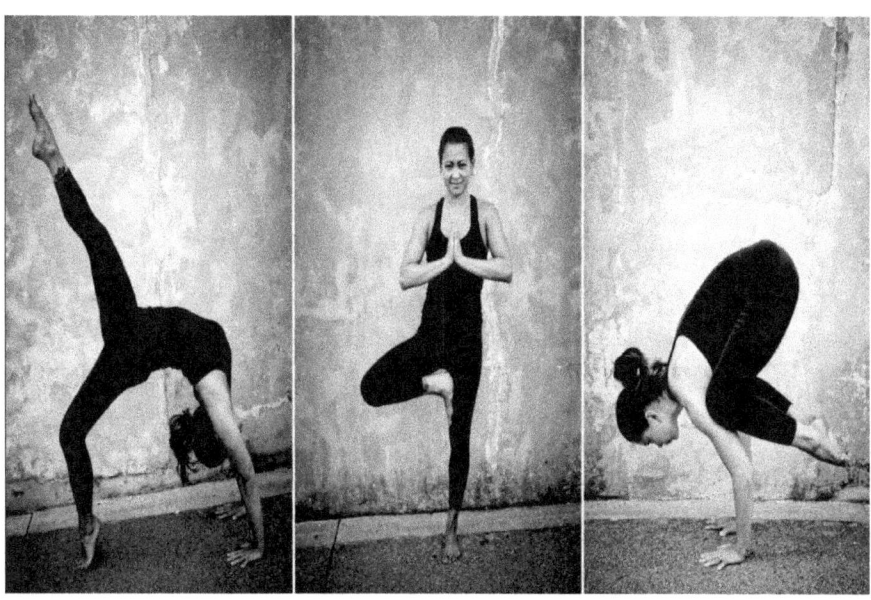

Plan

Leading by example: Women you need to hear this too!

Simple-minded: Men stop missing meals/eating too fast

Stuffing your face/splurging on weekends

Feast on salty foods/Drink all the time

Implement

Come on time; be prepared, keep quiet

Earn the right to talk, with hard work

Rest when you go home

Habit

Peace

Results

Physical Skills

Dancing, Yoga, Gymnastics, Martial Arts

Learn a little of each, stay culture

Take the stairs

To add strength to leg muscles and get a cardiovascular workout at the same time, try climbing plain old stairs. This can be done at home, in your office, apartment building, or on stair-climbing machines in the gym. Climbing two steps at a time is good for building the quadriceps (thigh muscles) and the gluteus (butt). Going down steps builds strength in the quadriceps and to a lesser extent, the hamstrings.

Weight training 101

Weight lifting "cold" can cause tiny tears in muscle tissue that you may not even be aware of at the time. Always do a five-minute warm up such as walk at a pace of at least 3.5 mph, ride a stationary bike or jump rope before lifting weights.

Exercise large muscles before smaller ones. When working the chest, back, or shoulders you are actually working groups of muscles. Working from large to small is more efficient. For example, you should do bench presses for the chest area before doing an exercise that isolates the triceps.

If you want to benefit from an aerobic workout too while weight training, try Super-Sets. This simply involves combining two exercises (not for the same muscle group) and performing one after the other with minimal rest. The continuous effort helps you achieve an aerobic state.

Can you feel the beat?

Depending on your age, level of conditioning, and your fitness goals, you should train in a particular heart-rate zone. Beginners should try to elevate their heart rate to 50%-60% of their maximum while intermediates and advanced should shoot for 70%-85% of their max. The higher your heart rate, the more calories you will burn and the more fit you can become. To figure your maximum heart rate, simply subtract your age from 220. For example, if you're 30 years old, you would have a maximum heart rate of 190. To work at 70% of your maximum heart rate, you would shoot for a heart rate of approximately 133 beats per minute (0.7 x 190). You can also count BPM (beats per minute) in 10-second increments and then multiply by six.

Tips on how to stick with your New Year's Resolutions

Focus on positive self-talk. Congratulate yourself every time you take a step towards your resolution goal. Seriously, pat yourself on your back or treat yourself to a massage.

Avoid berating yourself if you should fall back or break a resolution. Just brush yourself off and start over again.

Stick to your resolution by considering it a promise to yourself, not a test of your willpower.

Avoid situations that put you in temptation's path, meaning if you're on a diet, do not go to the ice cream parlor.

Keep a sticky note in a prominent place so that you see it every day, reminding yourself of your resolutions.

Be realistic. Make sure your plan is a realistic one that can fit into your lifestyle. Will you really have the energy to go out for that evening exercise class? (Then go in the morning). Make changes as easy and convenient as possible.

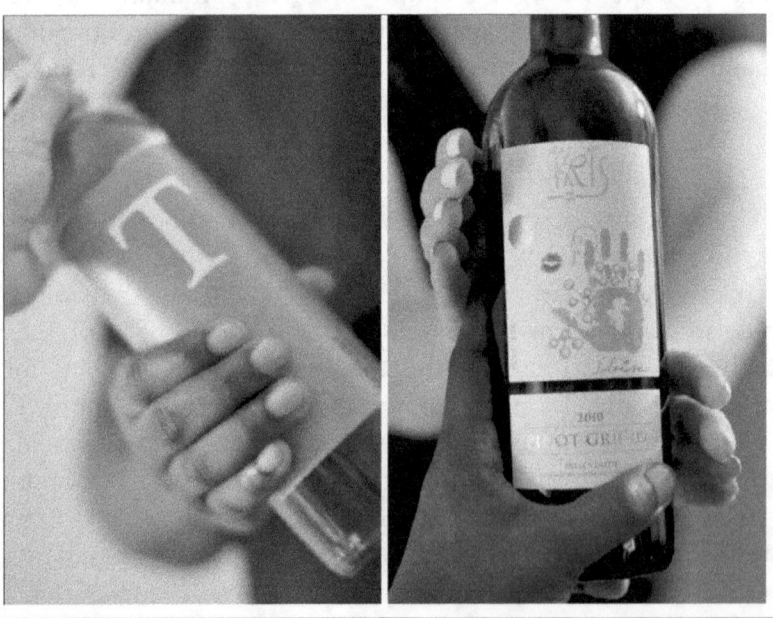

You can't talk about New Years without talking about…

Drinks & Drinks & Drinks & Drinks!

Alcohol can add hundreds of calories to your daily intake, which can make the difference between weight loss, maintaining your current weight, or gaining weight. A single glass of beer or wine can contain at least 100 calories. Having a few drinks 3-4 nights a week could be adding 1,000 unforeseen calories to your diet. On the surface it may seem like a fun night, but as your weight goals continue to falter you are going to have to consider making adjustments.

I meet so many people that are working out and literally drink the weight back on. They can't remember how many drinks they had and their inhibitions are lowered so they do not care. It takes them a while to realize they aren't seeing results because they are making the alcohol companies rich. If you work out during the week but drink heavy during the weekends you aren't letting your body rest. You're rewarding it with alcohol. How is that going to get you in good shape?

Alcohol also acts as an appetite stimulant, and can lead you to eat or crave foods that are not within your weight-loss plan. If you are dieting or are simply having trouble getting rid of that last little bit of fat, keep your alcohol intake to a minimum.

Easy Tips to Survive Events with Food and your Dignity

- Focus on talking to party guests and eating less. (Even better actually listen and learn something new.)
- Avoid hanging around the buffet table at social gatherings. (If you're starving you might not be able to resist.)
- Let people eat before you; maybe the unhealthy food will be all gone.
- Stick to high protein foods, fruit and veggies if given the choice. Go for the turkey, the sliced meats, the fresh fruit and raw veggies (without the dip).
- Avoid high fat hors d'oeuvres such as cheese, nuts, and saucy tidbits and fried anything. Instead, nibble on the veggies or chew gum.
- Eat before you go to a holiday gathering. Have a small meal such as fruit and low fat cottage cheese, yogurt or a low-calorie protein shake, a handful of grapes or an apple.
- Make yourself the designated driver at least half of the time. This will help you avoid calorie-laden alcoholic beverages.
- Instead of wine or mixed drinks, try soda water with lime and towards the end of the event, reward yourself for your good behavior with a glass of wine or your favorite drink.
- Bring your favorite low-fat recipe to an event or dinner. Then eat a lot of it (this proves it is good). Taste tempting treats but limit yourself to one small bite.
- Continue your workout schedule but ease off a bit to allow for the extra time holiday commitments take. You do not want to stress yourself out or quit exercising completely!

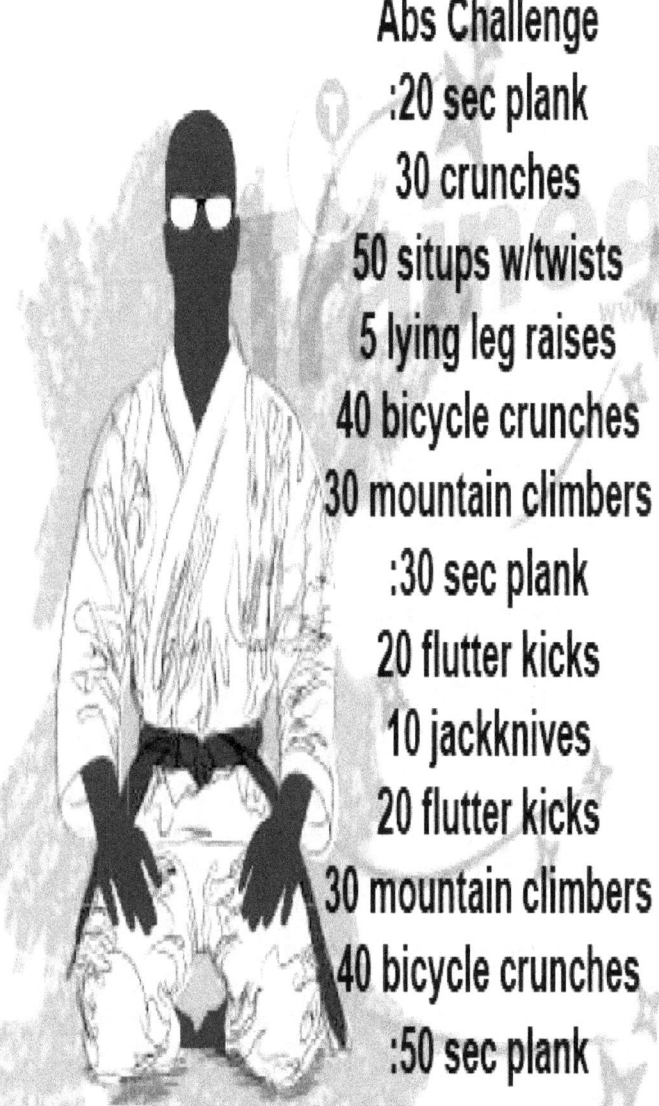

Abs Challenge
:20 sec plank
30 crunches
50 situps w/twists
5 lying leg raises
40 bicycle crunches
30 mountain climbers
:30 sec plank
20 flutter kicks
10 jackknives
20 flutter kicks
30 mountain climbers
40 bicycle crunches
:50 sec plank

theLifeSenSei.trainerze.com for the videos to exercises

Saying no to Mom or Dad

Ok you're going to your mother's house for a holiday meal; she gets insulted if you do not eat her "special dish." It's always fattening and she won't listen to you that you're trying to maintain your weight. It's a family tradition for you to gorge yourselves at meals and you know you're going to fall right into the trap. Here are some solutions.

Try a different tradition. Take your mother out for a change or go in with your other family members to have a healthy holiday meal at a park, a restaurant or someone else's home. Partner with family members to bring special low-fat treats to your mother's house if she insists on having the celebration there. Explain to her that you are each offering some alternatives to accompany her carefully and no doubt, lovingly prepared meal. Be assertive but appreciative of her efforts and help yourself avoid the trap! Good luck.

Being better prepared

Bringing your food to work is an excellent way to not only control what you eat but how much you spend. All it requires is a little bit of preparation on your part and smart shopping. You can buy in bulk and prepare your foods for the week, better yet make it a family affair over the weekend and enjoy yourself. Take the time to plan what type of snacks you're going to eat and make sure you bring some water as well.

Putting on weight

Gaining weight can be sometimes more difficult than losing weight. (Imagine that, someone is trying to gain weight?) But the same healthy eating habits and exercise regimes should apply. Aerobic exercise is what burns fat and uses calories. If you want to gain weight, you should cut back on aerobic exercise such as running and using machines or doing intense aerobic classes. Instead, concentrate on strength training with weights or through repetition. For aerobic exercise, swimming is a great all around body workout, as is power walking. These exercises, although aerobic, burn fewer calories than heavy aerobic exercise.

Eating Better

Eating right is as important to gaining weight as it is to losing it. Eat more frequently and choose more carbohydrates such as pasta, whole wheat bread and potatoes. Protein shakes help add bulk as do lean meats and nuts. Try eating a sandwich and a piece of fruit for a mid-morning snack and a handful of nuts for a mid-afternoon snack. A baked potato and a bowl of chili for carbohydrates are other good ideas. Fruit juices and whole grain cereals are also good choices for snacks. Be sure and eat five or six small meals a day. You do not need to add fatty or junk foods and sugary desserts to your diet to gain weight. Stick with high quality nutrient-dense foods. Cold sweet potatoes make great snacks and they are high in vitamins and fiber. Make your own fruit shakes with fruits, milk (ugh) and crushed ice.

The only reason you need a supplement to gain or lose weight is because you do not have the motivation or discipline yet. It is still in debate whether the products on the market actually make a difference compared to eating a healthy meal. For most people taking the supplements offers the feeling that you are doing the right thing. If you or someone you know needs that so be it. Just remember that a supplement isn't the real thing.

So what should we eat?

Eat what you want, and enjoy your life. The great rule is to burn more calories than you put into your body. If burning more calories doesn't work for you then try to eat healthier foods. If that doesn't work then make this meal plan work (tell them Sensei made you do it).

1. Eat six small meals a day, one every two to three hours
2. Eat a portion of protein and carbohydrates with each meal
3. Add a portion of vegetables to at least two meals a day
4. A portion is the amount of food approximately the size of the palm of your hand or your clenched fist
5. Drink at least 10 cups of water daily
6. Use performance nutrition shakes only if necessary to make sure you're consuming the nutrients you need
7. Plan your grocery list, and once a week have a day when you can eat conscience free

One song workout part 2

30 jumping jacks
10 squats
50 claws
20 pushups hands staggered
50 heel clicks
10 lunges with front kick
:30 sec plank with knees
30 jumping jacks

theLifeSenSei.trainerze.com for the videos to exercises

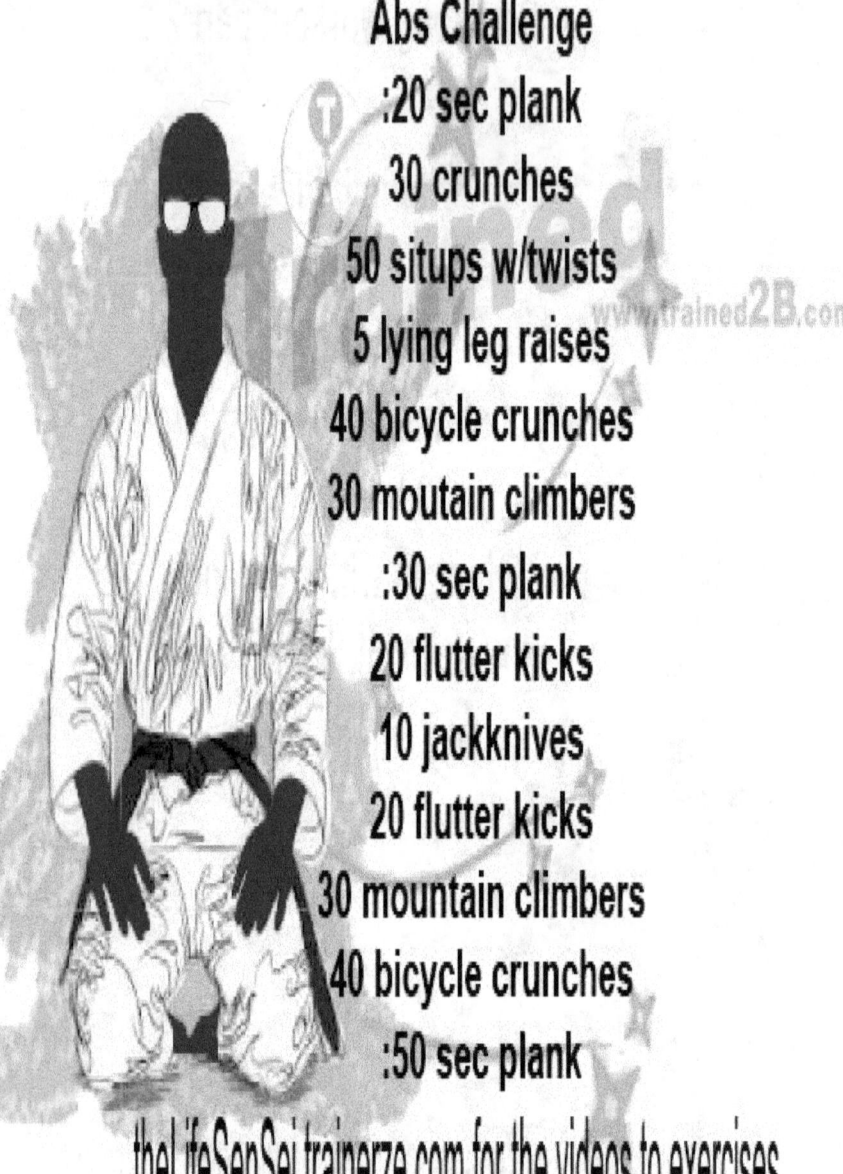

Abs Challenge
:20 sec plank
30 crunches
50 situps w/twists
5 lying leg raises
40 bicycle crunches
30 moutain climbers
:30 sec plank
20 flutter kicks
10 jackknives
20 flutter kicks
30 mountain climbers
40 bicycle crunches
:50 sec plank

theLifeSenSei.trainerze.com for the videos to exercises

the LifeSensei Workout Challenge

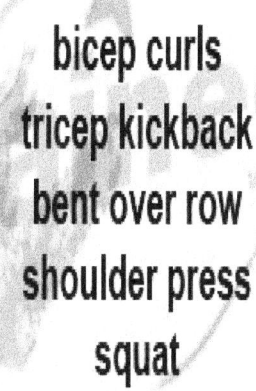

bicep curls
tricep kickback
bent over row
shoulder press
squat

:30 jumping lunges
:30 plank
:30 bicycles
in between each weight drill

theLifeSenSei.trainerze.com for the videos to exercises

Selected Bibliography

The Bible Old and New Testaments NKV –GOD

Brown, Carl. *The Law and Martial Arts (1998)*

Burner, David. *John F. Kennedy and a New Generation* (1988)

Cottrell, John. *Assassination! The World Stood Still* (1964)

Drinking Water - How Much? Factsmart.org web site and references

Food and Nutrition Board, National Academy of Sciences. Recommended Dietary Allowances revised 1945. National Research Council, Reprint and Circular Series, No. 122, 1945 (Aug),

Gentry, Clyde. *No Holds Barred: Ultimate Fighting and the Martial arts Revolution*. Milo Books. (2005).

"Harlem, the Village That Became a Ghetto," Martin Duberman, in *New York, N.Y.: An American Heritage History of the Nation's Greatest City,* 1968

Head, Tom. *The Absolute Beginner's Guide to the Bible*. Indianapolis, IN: Que Publishing, 2005

Homberger, Eric (2005). *The Historical Atlas of New York City: A Visual Celebration of 400 Years of New York City's History*. Owl Books

Howard, David (2002). *Outside Magazine's Urban Adventure New York City*. W. W. Norton & Company

Levitz, Maurey *What's In A Name? How the meaning of the term karate has changed*, New Paltz Karate Academy, Inc. (1998)

Mahan, L.K. and Escott-Stump, S. eds. (2000) *Krause's Food, Nutrition, and Diet Therapy*. 10th edition.

"Need for Harlem Theater," by Jim Williams, in *Harlem: A Community in Transition,* 1964.

NYC.gov – official website of the city

National coalition of domestic violence visit ncadv.org

Obesity in America.org

Plotz, David (November 11, 1997). "Fight Clubbed.

Reid, Howard and Croucher, Michael. *The Way of the Warrior-The Paradox of the Martial Arts" New York. Overlook Press: 1983.*

Research debunks health value of guzzling water. Reuters, April 2008.

Shigeru, Egami. *The Heart of Karate-Do.* (1976).

Shils *et al.* (2005) *Modern Nutrition in Health and Disease*, Lippincott Williams and Wilkins

Teen Dating Violence Information Guide. New York State Office for the Prevention of Domestic Violence. March 15, 2009.

Teen Dating Violence: What Parents Need to Know. Massachusetts Medical Society. March 15, 2009.

USDA National Nutrient Database for Standard Reference Search by Food

USDA National Nutrient Database for Standard Reference Nutrient Lists Search By Nutrient

Wookieepedia: The *Star Wars* Wiki — a wiki devoted to Star Wars

StarWars.com The official *Star Wars* website

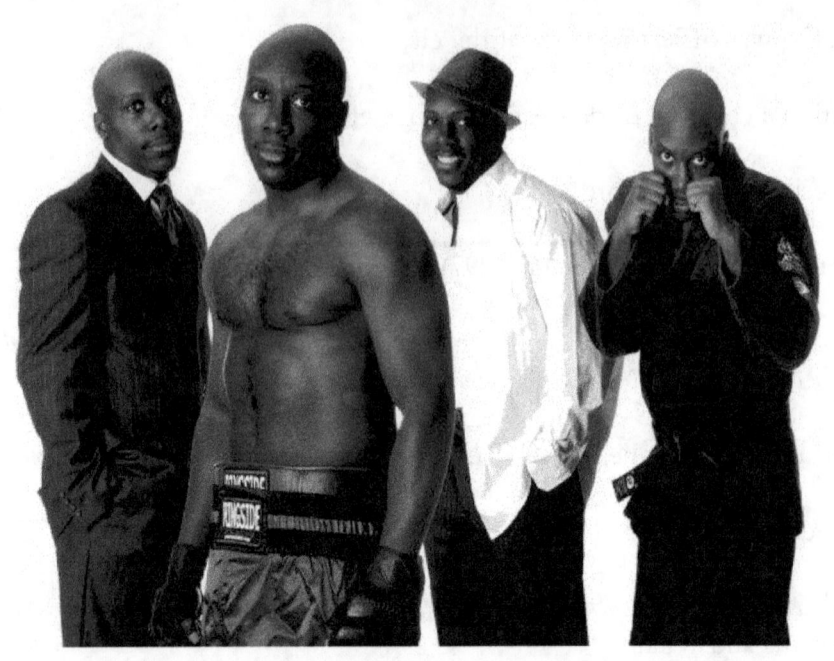

For More Information on Terence Mitchell

http:// Trained2b.com

http:// Artisticjournalist.com

Instagram handle: artisticjournalist

Twitter.com/#!/artisticjournal

http:// Youtube.com/user/Trained2b

http:// Facebook.com/ LifeSensei

http://Terencemitchell.bodybyvi.com/

Take my 90 Day Challenge with my shakes and supplements

http:// TheLifeSensei.trainerize.com

Online + Mobile Personal Training with New Videos,

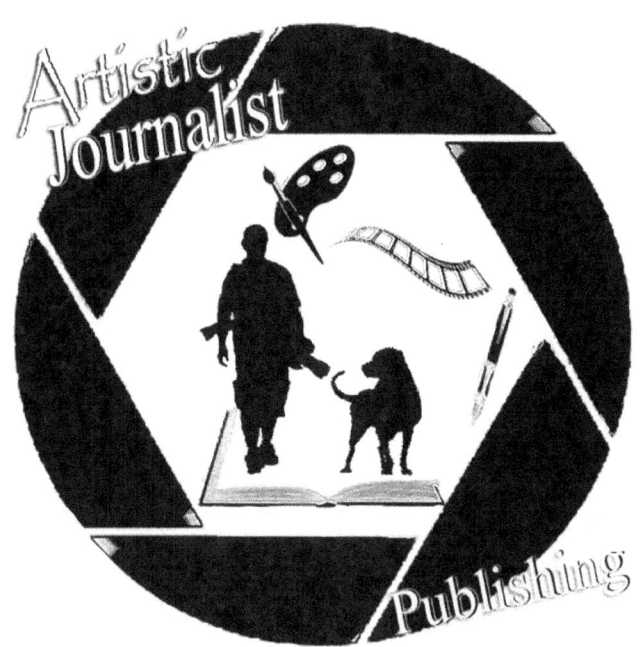

The Artistic Journalist

&

Artistic Journalist Publishing Present:

Life Sensei's Trained Subway Map Book Series

A Kids specific version

A Relationship specific version

A Spiritual specific version

A Martial Arts specific version

A Health specific version

Including Goals, Q + A, New Trained 2 B tips

www.ingramcontent.com/pod-product-compliance
Lightning Source LLC
Chambersburg PA
CBHW072208290526
45794CB00004B/1696